POST NATAL CARE

A Textbook for Midwives and Health Visitors

Nester Kadzviti Murira

Acknowledgements

I am indebted to postnatal mothers I have had the opportunity to care for and who were willing to share their experiences with me. I thank the midwives and obstetricians I have been privileged to work with in the provision of postnatal care services.

Foreword

Every woman who has carried a pregnancy has a unique story to tell about her experiences. There is no common experience. Each pregnancy and outcome has its own script no matter how often one falls pregnant. Unfortunately these experiences are usually compiled and generalized by health care providers, according to commonly identified phenomena of the experiences. The uniqueness of each woman's experience is lost in the process and the exceptions to these generalizations loose significance.

This book is based on observations and interviews of primiparous women in the first week of the postnatal period in a quest to understand the events surrounding, influencing and affecting primiparous women in the post natal period. The postnatal period, is a crucial period in which many women are exposed to ill health and some women remain with chronic ill health while some may loose their lives. This book draws attention to specific issues surrounding this very important but often sidelined phase in women's reproductive health and takes into consideration the fact that post natal events almost always have an impact on subsequent pregnancies and the woman's health as a whole.

In this book, women's knowledge, attitudes, practices, and how women cope with postnatal experiences are discussed. Women's risk perception in the postnatal period is explored. The community teaching, values and practices and their impact on the health of newly delivered women and their babies are explored. The experiences of women and the women's knowledge and expectations of the puerperium, their self-care skills are observed and documented. The reproductive health problems that women encounter in the postnatal period are highlighted. The post natal period is discussed according to phases for purposes of attention to events occurring within these specific phases and the impact they may have on a woman's health.

Nester Murira

Author

CONTENTS

This book explores the role health personnel can play in supporting women during the postnatal period.

Objectives

This book is designed to assist midwives and health visitors to:

- Provide appropriate care for women and their babies post delivery
- Make relevant life-saving observations of women post delivery

- Identify sources of morbidity and/or mortality postnatally

- Assist women to increase risk perception in the postnatal period

- Manage post partum haemorrhage efficiently in the third stage of labour

- Manage women's pain and discomfort efficiently post delivery

- Observe women closely in order to diagnose development of puerperal psychosis early

- Manage bereavement satisfactorily

- Advise new parents on general baby care skills

- Perform a thorough examination of the new born

- Assist new mothers and their support systems to develop safe and relevant postnatal self-care skills

- Advise new mothers on family planning methods of their choice

- Advise mothers on appropriate post natal exercises

- Respect women's culture while offering postnatal care

- Collect relevant evidence that can be used for improving post natal care services

CHAPTER 1

THE IMMEDIATE PUERPERIUM

The post natal period is the period immediately after the birth of the child and up to forty-two days post delivery. The first week of life is recognized as the most dangerous time for an individual in the developing world in the first 40 years of his or her life (James et al.,1987). This book pays special attention to events in the first week of the puerperium supported by evidence. There is little research in the postnatal period compared to research in other phases of the child bearing period, suggesting that the period is less valued by researchers and clinicians hence the low level of interest in the period (Rudman et al., 2008).

Women and their newborn babies and their families need a service that is individualised to address their physical, psychological, emotional and social needs (Richens,2007). Women also need a culture sensitive postnatal service that offers humane care and respects their dignity, views, beliefs and values of their partners and families in relation to their care and the care of the newborn babies.

Women should be fully involved in planning their care and be fully informed about relevant information and the advantages of a postnatal contact to enable them to be informed, confident active participants in their care. Women should be informed at each stage of care of the interventions that the woman and her newborn baby are exposed to. Information on the support available during this period should also be made available.

The immediate puerperium begins with events immediately following the delivery of the baby to the first twenty-four hours after delivery. The third stage of labour is the period from the birth of the baby to the delivery of the placenta.

The third stage of labour

Clinical expertise is an important component of clinical decision making and must be supported by evidence (Haynes,2002a). It is therefore important that midwives do not just rely on expert advice and personal beliefs and experience to guide practice, but must be supported by systematic reviews.

Based on evidence from systematic reviews, intramuscular oxytocin is a better uterotonic drug than syntometrine in the control of haemorrhage in the third stage of labour. Oxytocin reduces post partum haemorrhage without adverse effects (Cotter,2001; NICE,2007).

After delivery of the baby, immediate cord clamping reduces neonatal blood volume and red cell volume and may have other adverse effects on the baby as compared to delayed cord clamping (Hutton & Hassan, 2007; McDonald & Middleton,2008; Rabe et al.,2008). Early cord clamping in term babies was reported to reduce the incidence of jaundice while in preterm babies it increases the need for blood transfusion (Rabe et al.,2008). Cutting of the cord by the father of the infant promotes a strong bond between the father and child.

Expulsion of the Placenta

Care must be taken that the third stage of labour is actively managed to prevent haemorrhage. All blood on delivery of the placenta must be collected into a receptacle to be measured. The placenta and membranes must be examined before disposition. Retained membranes can cause serious haemorrhage and later puerperal sepsis. An oxytoxic drug must be given and pads checked in the case of retained membranes. Exploration of the uterus under anaesthesia must be done in the case of retained lobe. Retained lobe is a major cause of severe post partum haemorrhage and puerperal sepsis.

Haemorrhage

Haemorrhage is one of the leading causes of maternal mortality in the world and in Africa in particular (Udoma et al., 2003; Cochet et al., 2003; Yanagisawa & Wakai, 2008; Munjanja et al, 2007; Arowojolu, 2003; WHO, Safe Motherhood, 2006). Bleeding post delivery is heaviest during the first hour when the placenta has just separated from the uterine wall, uterine blood vessels are still open and the uterine muscle, the "living ligatures" are contracting to control the haemorrhage. Women are more likely than any other time to lose large amounts of blood with life threatening consequences within this period. A combination of complications of the third stage of labour, lack of resuscitation facilities, poor manpower skills, poor communication facilities such as telephones, and poor transport system to transfer clients in emergencies to well equipped health facilities, contribute to high maternal mortality rates in some developing countries(Mbizvo,1993).

In remote rural areas lives are lost unnecessarily because deliveries may be done by untrained birth attendants without means for control of haemorrhage, facilities for resuscitation are inadequate in the rural clinics in the developing countries, at primary care level health care staff may not be adequately trained to resuscitate women and infants in acute emergencies.

Haemorrhage exposes women to morbidity and mortality by the nature of its severity and especially where skills in managing it are lacking.

Where the tone of the uterine muscle is good, the haemorrhage may be controlled immediately by the uterine muscle action. Control of haemorrhage by the uterine muscle 'the living ligatures', may be slow where uterine muscles have been subjected to strain due to:

- Prolonged labour caused by uterine inertia
- Obstructed labour in mal-presentation
- Grand multiparity
- Macrosomia
- Polyhydraminous, and
- Multiple pregnancy.

In the circumstances above, there is need to compliment uterine action by giving oxytocic drugs until control of haemorrhage is achieved and the uterus is well contracted.

Active management of the third stage of labour which includes controlled cord traction, and the use of oxytocic drugs, has been found to reduce the length of the third stage of labour, maternal blood loss and the incidence of post partum haemorrhage as compared to expectant management of blood loss (Jangsten,2005). Active management of the third stage has been associated with an increased risk of nausea and vomiting and raised blood pressure especially where ergometrine is used. Such negative effects of haemorrhage control may be avoided through the use of alternative drugs with more pleasant effects. Expectant management of labour, or natural management allows the natural separation and delivery of the placenta.

A sudden gush of blood loss when the woman changes position to sit up or stand up for the first time post delivery may come as a result of the change of position, from lying in bed and the reason may be that blood could have been welling up in the uterus as the uterine muscle contracts to control the bleeding.

It is important to monitor the client closely and the texture of the uterus should be checked half hourly for the first two hours then hourly for subsequent two hours and four hourly thereafter to diagnose atony of the uterus early and take appropriate action.

Post natal bleeding may come as a surprise to primiparous women who have not received antenatal education. Primiparous women can be alarmed by the post delivery bleeding especially the loss of large quantities of blood. Research has revealed that it is difficult for women to give a good description or estimation of the amount of blood loss and some women may have no perception of the adverse effects of the haemorrhage.

Women may want to compare the post natal bleeding with their usual monthly period and their anxiety levels may rise as indicated by some women's comments below.

A.*'It is a heavy and an ongoing menstrual period. My mother said it is ridding of the blood that had been accumulating for the past nine months of pregnancy.'*
B.*'The flow is heavier than my usual monthly period; it seems that the pattern of my monthly cycle has changed.'* (Murira ,2010).

Signs of severe blood loss are:

- Restlessness followed by severe weakness
- Rapid thready pulse and low blood pressure.
- Parlour of skin which is easily noticed in the mucosa of the mouth, the tongue, palms and nail beds in dark skinned people and on the face in light skinned people.
- Breathlessness and sighing respirations
- The skin may become cold and clammy
- The client may faint or collapse

Control of haemorrhage

Quick action must be taken to control the haemorrhage.

- Appropriate action such as replacement of lost fluids by the use of an intravenous line.

- The source of the haemorrhage must be quickly identified by inspection of the tone of the uterus.
- Administration of an oxytocic drug must be done immediately if the cause of haemorrhage is uterine atony.
- Inspection of the birth canal for hidden tears and suturing of the tears must be done immediately.
- The loss of lives can be avoided by close monitoring of the women, immediate transfer of women to facilities with adequate resources for resuscitation.

Observations

- Blood pressure and pulse must be monitored closely every half hour for the first two hours, every hour for the following four hours and two hourly for four hours then four hourly thereafter for the first 24hours
- Blood pressure and pulse should be checked before transferring a mother into the postnatal ward and continued hourly for four hours then thereafter four hourly throughout the stay in the health facility until the woman is discharged home.
- Pad checks should be done hourly in the first two hours post delivery, then two hourly for four hours then four hourly thereafter.
- Close monitoring should be continued until the postnatal mother feels strong enough to be discharged from the unit.

Fundal Height

- The height of fundus may rise where there is internal bleeding due to atony of the uterus. Measures must be taken to contract the uterus by 'rubbing up a contraction' to activate the uterine muscle to contract or giving an oxytoxic drug.
- Fundal height measurement and uterine consistency should be observed hourly for four hours post delivery especially in clients likely to have postpartum haemorrhage such is multiparous clients, clients who have had difficult prolonged labour, clients who have had multiple deliveries and clients who have had surgical deliveries. Immediately post delivery, the consistency of the contracted uterus must feel like a tennis ball.
- A soft boggy or dough-like uterus is a sign of poor contraction and a cause for concern as control of haemorrhage is likely to be poor. Immediate action must be

taken to assist the uterus to contract using current measures according to management policy.

- After delivery, the height of the fundus is below the umbilicus and should continue to decrease until the uterus is no longer palpable around fourteen days post delivery. The fundal height should decrease by approximately one centimetre a day post delivery.

- The fundal height should therefore be measured on a day-to-day basis for the first fourteen days post delivery while the lochia is still flowing and active uterine contraction is still occurring.

Immediate Care of the mother

It is advisable to keep the postnatal mother in one place to enable her an opportunity to regain strength for at least an hour before moving her to a postnatal bed.

- Some women may feel thirsty after sweating profusely in labour. Women should be offered a cup of tea, a glass of fruit juice or water depending on what is available and the woman's preferences.

- Some women may feel extremely cold and may shiver uncontrollably due to the excessive sweating, loss of body fluids, and the body's reaction to the stress and exhaustion of labour.

- Women who have this experience may get immediate relief from a hot drink and extra warmth in the form of extra blanket or a heater.

- Some women may feel so exhausted that they prefer to be left alone and rest for a while. It is important to respect women's preferences post delivery.

Bladder Care.

The client must be encouraged to empty her bladder two hourly initially then four hourly to prevent over-distension of the bladder which interferes with uterine contraction and successful involution.

- The postnatal mother must be encouraged to take plenty of fluids to encourage the bladder to empty frequently by so doing regaining its tone.

- It is important to observe for hesitancy to empty the bladder and retention of urine which may occur where a woman has perineal trauma.

- Complaints of dysuria must be taken seriously and the woman should be tested for urinary tract infection.
- Perineal hygiene that emphasizes washing and wiping the perineal area from front backwards and change of pads two hourly and when the pad is soaked should be encouraged.
- Use of clean pads should be encouraged.

Communication

Women's preferences have to be identified and respected and a situation where women are managed routinely should be avoided at all costs.

- Client care must be client- centered respecting clients' preferences and choices in order to make the client as comfortable as possible.
- Good communication between the health care provider and the client is a very important principle of care that enables identification the client's choices and how she may be feeling.
- Individual attention must be paid to each woman and it is important to listen to clients' requests and attend to them to the best of one's ability and the facilities available.
- Talking to the client frequently and in a friendly manner creates a good atmosphere that enables the client to make requests and reports freely.

Client's comfort

- It is important that the client is comfortable and that she lies on a dry clean surface all the time.
- Some clients may request to take a shower immediately they feel strong enough to stand up, while some clients may need prompting to take a shower. It is important to constantly communicate with the client about her comfort.
- Semi-recumbent position is advisable to encourage pelvic drainage and full expansion of the lungs that assists in movement of the pelvic organs and ultimately pelvic drainage.

Perineal trauma

The perineum must be thoroughly inspected for bruises and trauma and appropriate decision made on managing the perineal trauma. Further exploration of the vaginal vault to exclude deep internal lacerations, and internal vaginal tears following instrumental delivery must be done. Such hidden injury may be a source of haemorrhage and may proceed to cause sepsis.

Complaints about discomfort in the vulval area must be taken seriously as tears and suture lines do not always heal as quickly as expected.

The client is advised on frequent vulval toilet to prevent odours and promote healing. Antibiotics may be prescribed where infection is likely to occur.

Perineal repair

The suturing or repairing of the internal lacerations and the perineum is best done immediately after the delivery of the placenta while the numbness and discomfort of delivery is still in place to allow the woman to accommodate all the discomfort at once and take it all as part of the delivery pain.

- The repair of the perineum should be done with as little discomfort as possible. Adequate local anaesthesia should be administered.

- Aseptic technique should be observed when suturing. Infection introduced during suturing may easily be transmitted to the internal organs of reproduction or become systemic because blood vessels are open and the genital system may have bruises enabling a quick entry of the infection into the circulatory system and body tissues.

- Suturing material must be well selected so that the deep fascia is sutured finely and in layers. Fine suturing material must be used bearing in mind that the perineum is a very tender area with soft thin tissue that rubs when walking or sitting and therefore can easily bruise.

- The superficial muscle layer and the skin must first be put in apposition and the apex of the wound identified before suturing occurs.

- Efforts must be made to bring the introitus back to its original shape to prevent undue pain to the client and promote quick healing.

- Suturing should be neat to avoid puckered and pleated perineal tissue, which may cause blister formation. Sutures should not be pulled tightly as they can cut through the tissues causing severe pain.

- Muscle and skin layers should be sutured separately to avoid gaping of the wound which may result in sinus formation and delayed healing causing unnecessary distress to the client.
- Suture ends must be cut short for the comfort of the client.

Perineal Complications

Episiotomies with a single layer of suturing have been observed in many primiparous women and the suture lines tend to break down very easily delaying the process of healing (Murira, 2010).

- A poorly sutured perineal area causes discomfort to the woman when she walks or sits. Poor sitting posture interferes with successful breast feeding.
- Perineal pain, like any other pain disturbs sleep leading to high levels of anxiety and exhaustion that may predispose a young mother to post natal depression. The client cannot position herself properly to feed her baby.
- Micturiction and defaecation can be so painful that a client may be hesitant to empty her bladder and bowel resulting in urine retention and constipation respectively.

Client Advice

- Advise clients to use soft, clean, and absorbent sanitary towels and keep the towels closed and in dust free packets.
- Clients should be encouraged to dispose sanitary towels every two hours or earlier where bleeding is still heavy.
- Clients are advised to wash the perineum clean with each change of sanitary towel or every two hours to avoid odours and to promote healing.
- Clients can be advised to use antiseptics, clean water or salty water to clean the perineal area.
- Washing the perineal area and wiping it dry must be done with each change of sanitary towel at least two hourly to promote quick healing and prevent infection and odours of the perineal wounds.

Anaemia

Anaemia following post partum haemorrhage has been reported widely and is a major cause of maternal morbidity. Iron deficiency due to blood loss is the most common cause of anaemia in the post partum period (Dodd et al, 2004).

Anaemia may easily be missed by health personnel on discharging women from health institutions especially where women leave the health institutions within the first twenty-four hours post delivery.

Women may not realize the consequences of haemorrhage and the subsequent anaemia unless they had prior information on how to identify anaemia. Women may report *'feeling weak, breathless, and fainting'*, but may not associate the way they feel with loss of blood. Health personnel should therefore make efforts to empower women throughout pregnancy and post delivery with information to prevent anaemia and to enable women to diagnose anaemia.

- Some women have associated the way they felt with other causes of stress and strain and weakness post delivery. Women have been reported to remark:
  'I feel faint; maybe it is because my baby suckles for a long time. It drains me.' (Murira,2010).

- Anaemia affects involution and delays repair of tissues post delivery.

- Women who have lost a lot of blood are generally lethargic, frail and tend to have a slow recovery post delivery.

- Anaemia causes debilitation in women post delivery and exposes them to heart failure and infections that may interfere with successful breast feeding, self-care and baby care.

- All women should have their haemoglobin checked before discharge from the postnatal ward.

Ambulation

Early ambulation post delivery is advised to prevent **thrombo-embolic complications and hypostatic pneumonia.** Not every woman is strong enough to walk around immediately post delivery. Each woman has to be assessed individually.

- Passive exercises and movement in bed must be encouraged for those women who must stay in bed for long periods because their conditions do not allow them to get out of bed early.

- Deep breathing exercises should be encouraged immediately post delivery to promote cardio-respiratory fitness and prevent hypostatic pneumonia (Hillsdon et al.,2005).
- Exercises must be continued throughout the postnatal period to tone up muscles relaxed by pregnancy hormones, reduce ankle oedema and reduce excessive weight gained in pregnancy.

Diet Post Delivery

Some postnatal mothers may not be ready to eat until a few hours after delivery. This could be because of extreme exhaustion.

Generally, post delivery women usually have a good appetite and may feel hungry more often than may be expected.

- Provision should be made for a cup of tea and snacks any time of the day as the women feel hungry and thirsty remembering that the woman is loosing essential body fluids and needs to replace them.
- A balanced diet should be encouraged immediately after delivery to promote tissue repair, speedy recovery and successful breast feeding.
- A high intake of fruit and vegetables provides vitamins essential for tissue repair, blood replacement and general recovery. Vitamins are essential for successful breast-feeding.
- The roughage contained in fruit and vegetables is essential in digestion as fillers and promotion of bowel movement preventing constipation.
- Appropriate advice on a diet rich in iron to replace lost blood must be continued throughout the postnatal period.
- The postnatal mother requires protein for tissue repair.
- Carbohydrates are essential in moderation for energy to enable the new mother to manage her new responsibilities.
- The postnatal mother requires minerals like calcium, potassium, magnesium not only for her personal needs but successful breast feeding and the needs of the new born baby.

Infection Control

The postnatal period exposes women to the risk of infection because of the presence of free flowing blood in the woman, raw wounds and bruises in the female genital system. Strict infection control measures must be observed to keep possibilities of infection to clients staff and the newly born infants.

Health personnel

It is of paramount importance that health personnel are not carriers of infection. Some measures that limit health personnel propelled infection are:

- Clean uniforms. Health personnel should ideally wear mufti until they reach their places of work then change into uniforms, shoes included. Once in uniforms health personnel restrict their movements within the hospital settings. This is a precaution taken to prevent bringing infection from outside environments into the hospital.
- Disposable aprons and gloves should be used once and disposed of before attending to the next client.
- Strict hand washing using recommended antiseptics should be observed and disposable wipes should be used.
- Health personnel with upper respiratory infections and diarrhoea, cuts and bruises to their hands as well as any other condition that can be transmitted should be prevented from working within the postnatal ward until they are cleared of the infection.

Aseptic Technique

- Aseptic technique, proper washing of hands, skin, and wounds should be done using recommended antiseptics and sterilised equipment.
- Care must be taken before performing procedures such as vaginal examination, examination of the newborn infant that thorough hand washing is done and gloves used to prevent direct contamination of raw areas which may cause internal infections.
- Equipment must be cleaned and autoclaved before it can be used again.
- Beds must be cleaned using recommended antiseptics before use by a new patient.

Bed Linen

- Linen must be properly washed with recommended detergents, and ironed before use.
- Linen must be changed immediately when soiled and changed daily where it is not soiled.
- Proper disposal of dirty linen must be observed to prevent mixing infected linen with uninfected linen. Infected linen must be bagged and washed separately.

Hospital Utensils

- Utensils must be collected timely from the client's bedside and washed immediately to prevent breeding pests like cockroaches, rats and flies which transmit disease.

Clients Food

- Clients' food must be fresh and well prepared in a clean environment to prevent food poisoning.
- Left over foods on the patient's bedside must be disposed of after every meal.

The Environment

- Floors and all surfaces must be washed and wiped with antiseptics to clean the surfaces of dust and dust- borne micro-organisms.

Disposal of wastes

- Surgical wastes such as bandages, swabs, specimens, that is all wastes that contain body fluids and items that have been used on clients such as aprons and gloves must be disposed of separated from household waste and incinerated.
- Sharps must be disposed of separately in special sharps buckets to prevent needle prick infections. When the bucket is full it must be sealed and incinerated.

Health care professionals must be vigilant and on the alert so that women and their newly born babies are not exposed to numerous postnatal complications. It is important that health personnel ensure that postnatal women have relevant professional support and can easily access health care services in the event of emergencies.

References

1. Cochet,L; Pattison,R.C; Mcdonald,A.P. Severe acute maternal morbidity and maternal death audit-a rapid diagnostic tool for evaluating maternal care. South *African Medical Journal*76, 2003; 93: 700-702

2. Cotter,A; Ness,A; Tolosa,A.(2001) Prophylactic oxytocin for the third stage of labour. Cochrane Data base System Rev.2001 (4): CD001808

3. Dodd, J; Dare, M.R; Middleton, P.Treatment for women with post partum iron deficiency anaemia. *The Cochrane database of Systematic Reviews*: John Wiley and Sons Ltd, 2004(4). Chichester, UK.

4. Haynes,R.B.Clinical expertise in the era of evidence-based medicine and patient choice. American college of physicians(ACP) Journal Club 2002a:136:11-4

5. Hutton,E, Hassan,E.S. Late versus early clamping of umbilical cord in full term neonates-systematic review and meta-analysis of controlled trials. JAMA 2007(297)(11) 1241-52.

6. James,M.L;Hudson,C.N.;Gebski,V.J. et al., An evaluation of planned early postnatal transfer home with nursing support. The Medical Journal of Australia,1987 Vol.147 pp434-438.

7. Jangsten, E; Strand, R; Gomez de Freitas, E et al., Women's perceptions of pain and discomfort after childbirth in Angola. *African Journal of Reproductive Health,* 2005; 9 (3):148-158

8. Mbizvo,M.T; Fawcus,S; Lindmark,G et al., Maternal mortality in rural and urban Zimbabwe: social and reproductive factors in an incident case-referent study. *Social Science and Medicine,* 1993; 36 (9):1197-205

9. McDonald, S.J, Middleton,P. Effect of timing of umbilical cord clamping of term infants on maternal and neonatal outcomes. Cochrane Database System 2008 Rev.16(2)CD004074

10. Munjanja,S.P. Maternal and Perinatal Mortality Study. Ministry of Health and Child Welfare Zimbabwe, 2007.

11. Murira,N. Communicating Sexual and Reproductive Health messages: In search of a model to increase risk perception among primiparous women in Zimbabwe. PhD

Thesis, (2010), Centre for Health and Social Care Research. Birmingham City University, UK.

12. NICE. Intrapartum care: care of healthy women and their babies during childbirth. NICE2007.

13. Rabe, H; Reynolds G; Diaz-Rosello, J. A systematic review and meta- analysis of a brief delay in clamping the umbilical cord of preterm infants. Neonatology (2008) 93 (2):138-44.

14. Richens,Y. Implementing the NICE guideline on postnatal care. The British Journal of Midwifery,2007,6(7) 412-417

15. Rudman, A; El-Khouri, B; Waldenstrom, U. Evaluating multi-dimensional aspects of postnatal hospital care. *Midwifery*, 2008; 24: 425-441

16. UNFPA *Maternal Mortality Update: Expectation and Delivery: Investing in Midwives and others with midwifery skills,* 2006. UNFPA Technical Support Division.

17. Udoma, E.J; Ekanem, A.D; John, M.E; Ekanem, A.I. The role of institutional factors in maternal mortality from obstructed labour. *Global Journal of Medical Sciences*, 2003; 57: 2 (1):13-17

18. Yanagisawa, S; Wakai, S. Professional healthcare use for life-threatening obstetric conditions. *Obstet Gynaecol*, 2008; 28(7):713-9

Chapter 2

DOMICILIARY POSTNATAL CARE

Domiciliary postnatal care is an organised professional health care service in the client's home in order to provide continuity of health care services after a client has left the formal health institution at the end of a pregnancy. Postnatal home visits should be an inaugural part of postnatal health care services made available to all new mothers especially primiparous women.

The Aim

The domiciliary postnatal care service aims at reducing maternal and infant mortality and morbidity following discharge from hospital and until the client recuperates from the effects of labour or gynaecologic ailment.

Specific Objectives

The postnatal domiciliary service is intended to:

- Enable the newly delivered women to access health care supervision and health care promotion advice.
- Give the new mothers confidence in their new roles and makes it possible for health personnel to make early diagnosis and prevention of complications.
- **Reduces morbidity and mortality**
- **Improve the quality of life** for the mother and baby in particular, and the health of her family as well.
- **Assist clients with known health problems** to cope in the home environment
- **Monitor the clients' recovery** in order to identify occurrence of puerperal abnormalities early and manage them accordingly.
- **Support and build confidence** in new mothers to adjust to their new roles as mothers given their socio-economic status and environment
- **Equip mothers** with self-care skills to enable them to participate fully in their care
- **Equip mothers** with baby care skills

- **Provide health promotion** information to mothers and their families
- **Motivate new parents** and advise on family planning
- **Create awareness** in the mothers of how their bodies work
- **Empower couples** with adequate information to enable them to identify abnormalities to their health and the health o their offspring and seek help without delay
- **Refer women** with special needs to relevant institutions and organizations.

Domiciliary Post natal care **consists of planned activities** of care to cater for the health needs of the whole woman and not just her reproductive system. This includes **assessment of psychological, social, physical, environmental and economic** status and how they impact on the woman's health as well as strengthening relevant caring skills.

Planning a Postnatal Visit

Priorities

Clients with known health problems should be seen earlier than other clients in order to assist them to settle smoothly at home post delivery otherwise all women are entitled to domiciliary care as a part of health care and reproductive health in particular.

- Home visits are best made two to three days after a client has left a health institution. This enables the health care staff to assess the condition of the mother and child in their natural environment based on the client's condition on leaving hospital.

- Visiting the client two or three days after leaving the continuous care of health care staff gives a new mother ample time to observe her baby, assess her self care skills and baby care skills and identify areas of concern and her information needs. Women are happy to know they can access help anytime and help can come to them as expressed by one primiparous mother below.

"It is wonderful to know that you can get such a service. If I should have problems this early after delivery, I cannot imagine myself going to see the doctor in my state. I don't want to have to go and queue at the doctor's rooms for hours in my first week after delivery Queuing for a service in my state is very distressing. I don't like the idea of packing nappies, wipes, you name it, to get ready for a nappy change in a crowded doctor's room. And how do I get there? It means I have to pack a bag of baby stuff, walk to the nearest bus stop with package and bundle in hands, and wait indefinitely at the bus stop for

a crowded bus. By the time I get into the city centre my legs are numb. My breasts are weepy. My baby is yelling. I am boiling hot. The stitches down my bottom burn. What if the episiotomy opens? It means I have to pad myself with as many sanitary towels as possible to prevent the "feminine accident". Very few women are lucky to have stopped bleeding by the first week. There is nothing as embarrassing to a woman as messing up your dress! I still have to walk another kilometer and a half to the doctor's rooms. It is not always that you have extra money for a taxi. Imagine the chaffing and discomfort of four pads between your legs as you try to walk! Doctors don't know some of these hidden discomforts. Most of them are men! Even the women doctors have become men in thinking, by association of course." That's one side of the issue. What do a I wear to go to the doctor's? I still bear witness to a cow-size appetite I had developed in the last few months of expecting. My tummy could pass for a six months pregnancy! This is a wonderful service.'(Murira,2010).

Discharge Planner

This is a comprehensive report that coordinates client care beyond the hospital setting. It is generated from the institution where the postnatal mother is discharged to the community team who will take care of the domiciliary care.

- The discharge planner communicates client information to the team/agency/institution assuming responsibility for continuing care of the client.
- It contains information on the client's condition and her care needs to enable continued care
- It facilitates assessment of the client's condition by the receiving team.
  The advantages of this approach are that:
  Advice and education are not blindly given but are personalized and objective.
- Realistic assessment of the client's constraints and available resources including environmental factors can be made.
- The client is in control on familiar ground in her home. She can converse freely in a relaxed manner and ask questions she may not be free to ask in hospital.
- It enables a realistic assessment of the client's resources and the help she requires.
- It enables health personnel to give relevant advice that is responsive to the individual client's needs and the resources available to her.

Preparation for a home visit

Referral system should be clear and relevant specialist services should be in place and accessible to clients. The health visitor must be well equipped for the visit. She must have the following equipment:

A sphygmomanometer,

A stethoscope,

A tape measure,

A thermometer,

Portable baby scales,

Baby milestones books,

Dressing packs,

Antiseptics,

Relevant health information leaflets for both mother and baby

Family planning kit with a variety of the available oral and barrier contraceptives.

The Health Visitor

A health visitor is a trained member of the health team who provides health care services, health education, health promotion as well as environmental advice to health care clients within the client's home.

- The health visitor is a part of the continuous care community health care team who provides a link between the health care teams in health institutions and the community.
- The health visitor is the link that ensures that clients are continuously monitored, have access to health care teams and can access help when they need it.
- The health visitor therefore is a good communicator and team player who can quickly assess a client, make a quick decision on where and when they should call assistance of other professionals or refer a client for specialist care.
- The health visitor is familiar with the health care system and the referral system to enable smooth transfer of clients from the community to the health institutions and specialist services when the need arises.
- The health visitor has skills in planning and organizing her work independently.

- She/he has skills in counselling, and patient teaching.

- She/he is familiar with clients' culture, the customs and beliefs of the community she/he serves so that she/he can incorporate these in client teaching (Leininger & McFarland,2005).

- She must understand family dynamics, which is important in the support of the new mother.

- She/he must be open minded to enable her to deal with the varied situations she comes across in the homes (Edelman & Mandle,2005)

Approaching the Client

Before the client leaves health institution, it is important that the client's address after leaving the health institution is known by the health team to enable a visit by the health visitor.

Demographic information of the client to include her name, parity, and brief history of her condition, the type of delivery she had, the underlying condition and relevant information about the baby's condition at delivery and on leaving the health facility should be on the discharge planner. **This information forms the baseline data of the care plan** and the advice. It helps the community team to assess for improvement, deterioration or development of complications in the client.

- Clients with known problems such as single parents, those who have had difficult labour and those whose babies need close monitoring should be seen earlier than other clients in order to assist them to settle at home as smoothly as possible.

Uniqueness of a client

- Each client is a unique individual. Each woman's social environment and sources of support and her personal circumstances are unique.

- Every woman must be managed as an unique individual. No two women are similar in their needs, feelings, and expectations.

- Babies too must be considered as unique individuals. Babies do not necessarily have to resemble any other person in appearance, developmental milestones and behaviour. In some families a new mother may be taken to task by relatives or spouse because they believe the baby must resemble someone in the family.

- Every client has skills no matter how basic. It is up to the health care provider to identify these skills through observation and discussion and recognise these skills as a basis for advice, improvement of self care skills, emotion handling and promotion of compliance with any new skills and information the health visitor may introduce.

- Clients are influenced and affected by the environment in which they live. The health care provider can only be exposed to these influences through creating a trusting relationship with the client and obtaining information through good interviewing skills. That way the health personnel will be able to understand the client well, empathise with her, and together formulate a care plan that is comfortable for the client.

Clients desire to recuperate quickly and live healthy lives. Health personnel should however appreciate that when clients do not achieve this goal, there is usually an underlying problem beyond their control that the health personnel should try to assess and investigate to assist the client to achieve as quick a recovery as possible.

The Social Context

The client lives in an environment that impacts on her way of life positively or negatively. It is important to pay attention to this environment as it is inseparable from the client.

The health visitor assesses the environment throughout the visit to get a clear insight of some of the constraints a mother may have or some advantages some mothers may have in self care and baby care. Such information helps to select appropriate approaches to care and in offering relevant advice that is not removed from the client's way of life.

Economic Status of the new mothers

Women may have challenging circumstances post delivery and these challenges become clear to health personnel only through home visits.

Ms. Rose delivered a baby girl and was sent home from hospital after twenty four hours. She was unemployed and a single mother. She lived with her parents. Her mother was breast feeding her seventh nine month baby boy. When the health visitor arrived to see Ms Rose and the baby Ms Rose was about to leave home for the city centre to a night club, to try and "raise the doctor's fees and the hospital fees", to use her words. She had not breast fed the baby since arriving from hospital. She did not want to encourage lactation, according to her mother. On examining her, Ms Rose had padded her breasts to prevent any milk leaks. She had packed her vagina with cotton wool to stop bleeding. The baby looked dehydrated and was crying uncontrollably most likely because of hunger.

Ms Rose was persuaded to breast feed her baby after a long discussion with the health visitor. She was supervised for three visits and referred to the social welfare services. Ms Rose and her baby were fortunate to have a health visitor coming to their rescue. There are many women and new born babies who meet with difficult circumstances after discharge from hospital and have no one to turn to because of lack of comprehensive health care services. Postnatal domiciliary services save lives.

It must be appreciated that there are many factors that affect the health of individual women and a large number of these are embedded in the environments around the individual women and traditions upheld by the individuals and the societies in which they live. If these factors are unknown to the health provider or are ignored and omitted in client education, health promotion and self care messages, women and their newly born babies can be greatly disadvantaged.

There are myths, beliefs, taboos and practices around the new mother some of which increase morbidity and mortality. The health visitor needs to identify and familiarise herself with the clients' beliefs and practices post delivery in order to help women promote their own health, desist from potentially harmful practices and be able to make informed decisions when their lives are exposed to potential danger. It should be remembered that whenever women are persuaded to stop a practice an effective alternative with convincing and scientific explanation should be provided .The individual's health beliefs, her social and economic status must be known to health personnel in order to help the individual make sound decisions and for health personnel to plan relevant and appropriate care for the mother and her infant.

Social Support

There are four types of social support that a new mother can have access to namely:

- Emotional support involving empathy, love and trust.
- Instrumental support involving practices that directly aid the person in need.
- Information support which involves provision of relevant information essential for managing personal and environmental problems and
- Appraisal support which is availability of information enabling self evaluation and evaluation of circumstances one finds herself in (Stein, 1997). Appraisal support enables one to make social comparisons.

Postnatal mothers may access emotional support from their spouses and immediate family but this should not be taken for granted. Members of the immediate family especially mature female members are usually at hand to provide instrumental support. Mature women also provide some form of information support but this depends on how well informed the sources of support are. It is important that health personnel are aware of the type of support a postnatal woman has access to.

There are important social factors that health personnel must note about social support. The first factor is the type of support provided and whether it is focused or general. Health personnel may assume that every new mother leaving a health institution will be able to access some support in the community. Observations have revealed that women do not always have access to adequate useful support in the communities. The second factor is the frequency of the support, whether it is continuous, sustained and therefore durable or whether it is sporadic. Some women may move in temporarily with relatives who can advise on self-care and assist with baby care in the first few weeks post delivery, but there are many young women who are at risk because they have to cope with the postnatal demands and challenges on their own. The third factor is the intensity of the support. The fourth factor is the person providing the support. These four factors determine the quality of the support offered.

Reproductive information, obstetric emergencies, the process of involution and the relevant life-saving support are not common knowledge in many households. The lives of many women are at risk in the postnatal period because essential life-sustaining support is not available. There are commonly accepted community beliefs and practices and housewives tales that have been accepted as the management of a postnatal mother but some of these practices can be life-threatening to a new mother and her baby. The perception of the person receiving the support (subjective factors) and the actual measure of the support by an onlooker or independent assessor are important in assessing quality of support offered (objective factors) may differ, young inexperienced women may be content with reassurances offered by their mentors while their lives are exposed to danger.

Women members of the immediate family in communities have been known to be sources of support to fellow women during the child-bearing phase in many societies hence women's culture is regarded as the caring culture (Stein, 1995). There is a belief that there is a relationship between one's health and the social support one gets especially in the child bearing phase. The perception of support in a woman is reported to lead to a sense of control (Stein,1997; Maimbolwa,2003). It has also been reported that women with close support in the perinatal period can easily be identified as they are usually free from anxiety and are well nourished (Stein, 1997; Hodnett, 2002).

The health visitor however must always be on the alert and not make assumptions about available support. Women and their carers must be exposed to evidence based information and practices that promote quick recovery and good health. The health visitor must explore commonly accepted practices, food taboos and advise on food combinations that form a balanced diet which is essential for postnatal mothers and promotion of good health in general. First time mothers almost always derive emotional support and informational support from their mothers and grandmothers. The health visitor must ensure that these sources of support are well informed and equipped with effective perinatal practices.

The health visitor should be able to advise sources of support on relevant areas that require comprehensive support in order to assist the new mother.

- The health visitor must pay special attention to providing evidence based information and skills support and to both the new parents and their sources of support.

- Special observation must be paid to cultural practices that interfere with quick recovery and promotion of good mother and child health.
- It is important that the health visitor assesses the type of support and quality of support a new mother is receiving from those close to her.
- It is important to assess the knowledge gaps displayed in the support, the prevailing practices and how they impact on the client's health and the health of the newborn infant.
- It is through this thorough assessment that the health visitor is able to plan health education, health promotion and an effective care plan for the client.

Primiparous Clients

- More time should be budgeted for visits to primiparous clients. An objective assessment of the client includes all aspects of self care skills as well as assessment of basic baby care skills.
- Information needs of primiparous clients are expected to be more than those of the multiparous client and yet the primiparous clients may not readily ask questions because she may not know what problems are likely to arise or what skills she may need in future.
- The health visitor has to probe and find out what information needs the client may have.
- The health visitor should engage in demonstration of skills and supervising skills learning.
- When visiting primiparous clients, it is best to enquire who she lives with and include this person in discussion of care and the relevant baby care skills. Primiparous women are targets of numerous and sometimes conflicting and confusing advice from relatives, inlaws, neighbours and friends.
- It is important that primiparous women are exposed to the correct information and the correct self care and baby care skills right from the outset. The presence of relatives may be an advantage in that what is discussed and taught may have a multiplier effect.

The Multiparous Client

- The multiparous mother is familiar with some events post delivery. It is best to find out how she has managed before, then the midwife can re-enforce or perfect current skills as well as update on new trends and make available relevant information.

- Some clients may be comfortable with their way of doing things that there is no need for the midwife to intervene unless her practices endanger the well being of the baby, or her own health.

- When a midwife suggests on an alternative method of self care or baby care skills, she should provide convincing information that supports her advice. The emphasis should be on providing well-informed advice and information, updating skills and providing safe techniques in self care and baby care.

- The health visitor must exclude potential sexual and reproductive complications associated with multiparous women such as:

- **High blood pressure**. Blood pressure must be closely monitored.

- **Haemorrhage.** The lochia must be checked on each visit to exclude post partum haemorrhage.

- **Anaemia.** Haemoglobin must be checked and any signs of anaemia are thoroughly investigated. Family planning advice must be given and advice on long term methods given. Dietary advice must be given.

- **Possible pelvic organ prolapse.** The woman is advised to take pelvic floor muscle exercises seriously to prevent pelvic floor muscle sagging, and prevent bladder control problems.

References

1. Edelman, C.L; Mandle, C. L. Health Promotion throughout the life span. 6th Ed. Mosby, 2006.

2. Hodnett, E.D. Pain and women's satisfaction with the experience of childbirth: a systematic review. *Am J Obstet Gynaecol Suppl*, 2002; 186 (5): 160-72

3. Leininger,M.M; McFarland,M.R. *Culture Care Diversity and Universality. A Worldwide Nursing Theory.* 2nd. Ed. Jones & Bartlett Publishers, 2006. London

4. Maimbolwa,M; Ahmed,Y; Diwan,V; Ransjo Arvidson, ASafe Motherhood Perspectives and Social Support for Primigravidae Women in Lusaka,Zambia. *African Journal of Reproductive Health,* 2003; 49 (3): 40-49

5. Stein, J. *Empowerment and Women's Health. Theory, Methods and Practice.* Zed Books Ltd, 1997. New Jersey.

Chapter 3

MEETING THE CLIENT ON DOMICILIARY VISIT

Visiting new mothers in their homes involves creating a relationship with the client as well as making a good impression on the client. Relationship is created through good communication. The health visitor is a stranger in a client's home and should therefore seek to be accepted first. It is important that health personnel adopt client centred approaches to communication preferably a collegial approach (Ellis, 1995). The client's rights, her needs and wishes take the centre-stage. Ethical and humane principles of respect, privacy and self-determination must be observed (Seedhouse & Lovette,1992; Hope et al., 2004). The client's culture must be respected(Leinenger & McFarland, 2006). This relationship is very important to enable exchange of information that forms the basis of client education and advice.

- Clients need to be informed of an intended visit by the health team and the purpose of the visit so that visits are made at a time that is convenient to the client and her family.

- The health visitor must understand that she/he is a guest in the client's home and must therefore show respect for the client and her family. Relationship with clients is a very complex construct. It requires the finest aspects of attributes.

- Good communication, confidence in performance of skills and display of knowledge is important. A good impression has to be displayed and sustained throughout the home visits.

Each health visitor should be familiar with basic guidelines for postnatal domiciliary care implementation such as:

- Development of a clear well documented individualised client care plan based on the discharge planner and the current condition of the woman. The care plan should take into consideration pertinent events of the woman's antenatal, intrapartum and immediate postpartum period (Richens,2007).

- Women should be given as much information as they wish to access about their health and the health of their babies so that they can develop confidence in self-care and the care of their babies. The signs and symptoms of potentially life threatening conditions to themselves and their infants and family should be pointed out and relevant information on relevant contacts given.

- Women should be given information of other services that they may wish to contact that contribute to the improvement of their health. Each woman should be given leaflets about her personal health and the health of her newborn infant.

- The health visitor should take note of the woman's physical and mental health and the social support available.

- The health of the woman and her newborn infant must be reviewed on each visit. Each woman's care plan should be reviewed at each contact.

- Recognition of skills in other health professionals and making prompt referrals should the health visitor be unhappy or unsure about the condition of the mother or that of her newborn baby.

- All health visitors should be well informed about postnatal care principles and ensure that they are up to date with knowledge and skills in communication, identification and management of clinical risk to assist women and their newly born infants.

Most health visitors are strangers to their clients on first visit. It is not often that the midwife who arranges the home visit is the one who visits the client. It is imperative for the health visitor to introduce herself to the client, if the client and the health visitor have not met before or she meets people she has not met before, she must spell out the objective of her visit. This helps to create rapport. Small talk, like comments on the whether or common current topic of interest can also be used to relax everyone present and initiate a conversation.

- On the initial visit to a client's home, the health visitor introduces herself to the client and her relatives in the home. She must state her name and the office in which she is based and spell out her objectives clearly. A business card, and contact telephone or information on how she can be contacted is essential information for the client to have. Clients, especially primiparous clients may want to contact the midwife frequently for queries and sometimes just to be reassured that all is well.

Obtaining Postnatal Information

Consent

Clients do not readily consent to and comply with what they do not understand. It is therefore necessary in any client-health provider encounter to start with a clear explanation of the   purpose of the visit, the advantages to the client, and what is expected of the client. In the event of procedures to be performed, these have to be clearly explained to the client as well as any risks associated with the procedure (Seedhouse & Lovette, 1992;Liley,2001).

Interviewing

- Interviewing postnatal mothers is an essential process in domiciliary postnatal care as it enables health visitors to collect essential information for development of a postnatal care plan. Interviewing may not always be a simple extraction of information a health visitor requires, but requires good communication skills(Lloyd & Bor, 2003; Heron,2001) Clients may be guarded and may resent intrusive and inquisitive in-depth interviews by a stranger discussing sexual and reproductive issues. It is important to understand the client's culture first and whether issues related to reproduction can be openly discussed. The subject of sexual and reproductive health is not openly discussed in some cultures, and this may affect the responses the health visitor may ask.

- Some responses may be brief and guarded. Clients make an assessment of the health visitor and decide on how much to tell and what to leave out. Clients can only disclose what they are willing to divulge. This is one of the limitations of an interview.

The age of the woman and the subject of reproductive health may affect women's responses.

- Interviewing women in their homes in particular where other members of the family are present may not be simple. Young women may not talk in the presence of their in-laws or other members of the family. Assumptions about the presence of relatives or spouses should not be made as some young women may not talk freely in the presence of their spouses. It is therefore necessary to obtain a verbal consent from the women for their spouses to be present during the interview. Curious family members can be politely asked to wait until they are invited for a discussion. Interviews are therefore best held in a private room away from other members of the family. This absence of the elderly women and in-laws yields good interview information.

- In the brief post natal contact with the postnatal mother, health personnel may not engage women fully in acquiring self-care skills post delivery and technical skills to assist them with the skills expected of a new mother. Through in-depth interviews and observations, women's self- care skills and cultural practices that are inherent in the communities around a new mother can be revealed. The health visitor must take this opportunity to offer evidence based advice to the new mother.

- The first week is an opportune time to assess the impact of community practices on the health of a new mother and newborn baby. It is imperative to document the attitudes, the beliefs, the practices around the new mother in the community as this information is crucial in making a postnatal care plan for the mother and developing appropriate interventions.

- Interviewing a postnatal mother should be done in a quiet environment with little or no disturbance. Interruptions by family members, laughter and comments, the television, a radio, or the baby's cry distract the client who may loose her trend of thought, and may withhold crucial information essential for her care.

- It is important to reduce the chance of being overheard because the client may hesitate to share confidential information.

- It is important for the health visitor to establish how the new mother thinks she has been coping since leaving hospital as such information gives the health visitor an insight of the problems the new mother has encountered.

Questioning Skills

- Questions should be open ended to allow the mother to express herself freely, tell her story, and take control of the interview (Wimpenny & Gass, 2000).

- The interview should be regarded as a process of sharing personal and intimate information that should be regarded as confidential in order to identify the client's problems (Newell, 1994). The interview therefore should be client -centred.

- Close-ended questions have very little room in a postnatal interview, as they do not yield much information to enable the midwife to help the mother (Polit & Hungler,1993;Bryman,2004). They shift the focus from the client to the provider. The midwife notes areas of concern and probes for more information if need be. If the mother seems to hesitate to state clearly some of her concerns, the midwife could probe by saying," You mean..."and wait for the mother to carry on.

- Where there is disagreement on certain issues young mothers may not freely point that out and the midwife may miss some of the queues.

If too many questions are asked the client may feel that the midwife wants to control the conversation and that may retard conversation. Some clients may then wait for the midwife's questions that will be answered by a 'yes' or 'no' answer.

Listening

The health visitor's attributes should include that of good listening skills. She should listen carefully and take note of non-verbal cues that she then uses to probe for more information. She could ask a simple question like," What do you mean?" to enable the client to express a gesture like shrugging shoulders.

- It is important not to rush the client. Rushing the client makes the client nervous causing the client to withhold some important information. Sometimes a client keeps quiet because she is looking for the proper word to describe what she wants to say or because she is recalling and reflecting on something.

It is important for the health visitor to take note of the tone of the client's voice and ascertain if it indicates anger, happiness, frustration, or unmet needs.

Assessment

Assessment is a process of getting to know the client in order to plan for her postnatal needs. Assessment is an important process to establish baseline information with which to plan an intervention and evaluation of care. The assessment lays the foundations for further management.

- Assessment must be holistic to include the environment, the social, mental and physical state of the client.
- Assessment involves three skills namely, observation, interviewing and physical examination.
- Both parties, the health visitor and the client should be active participants in this process. The client is engaged in the process of information giving to the health visitor. This is a part of problem identification, which provides leads to goal setting and problem solving. It enables relationship building which is essentially a communication process.
- Interaction between the health care provider and client is key to accessing the client's problem and for the client to get a detailed orientation of what support is on offer (Ley, 1990).
- The health provider, listens to what the client has to say about her condition, observes the skills the new mother has, explains physiological changes a client may wish to understand, and demonstrates new skills.

Observation

The home visit enables observation of both the physical settings in which postnatal activities take place and the human activities going on during this period. Observations of women in their natural environment is a powerful method of learning and gathering rich information and the observation can be used on its own or in combination with other data collection methods such as interviewing(Bryman, 2004; Ziervogel et al., 1997). Observations are referred to as a fundamental base of seeking behavioural and social information (Wolcott, 2005). Through the use of observations, one has the opportunity to collect first order data on the scene of the event where one can personally see what is taking place.

- Observation increase understanding of a phenomenon and opportunities to verify the meanings of what is observed. Observations can be used therefore to confirm information collected (Bryman, 2004; Ziervogel et al., 1997). Validation of the events occurring around the mother can be realised through agreement between the health visitor and the mother (Adler & Adler, 1994). Being with the postnatal woman for a length of time in the client's home in the first week post delivery enables observation of the practices that may impact negatively on the health of the woman (Wang et al.,2008).

- The observations enable the health visitor to decide how to assist the woman and the communication model the health visitor can adopt (Tenant,2002;Timmermans et al.,2005)

There are three types of observations a health visitor can make namely:

- Descriptive observations in which the observer collects details of every aspect of the events (Angroseno & Mays de Perez, 2000). This type of observation is involving and generates lengthy notes. It is ideal in postnatal care but the health visitor may spend a lot of time recording irrelevant information. The health visitor needs to be a good observer picking on **issues likely to interfere with the health** of the mother and baby.

- Focussed observation ignores certain things classified as irrelevant and describes a particular phenomenon of interest only. Selective observation enables an observer to concentrate on chosen activities of concern like the state of breasts, perineal area and general application of self-care skills. This type of observation is ideal in postnatal research. The intention of postnatal observation is to glean information that is used to provide holistic care. Focussed observation has a role in postnatal observations.

- The third type of observation that uses a check list to be ticked after observation may not be useful in observing behaviours and skills.

The clinician's position in a home visit can fluctuate between a complete observer and a participant- observer. The position of a complete observer can be taken when the observer does not have to participate in any activity around a woman whereas the observer becomes a participant- observer when involved with the activities going on as well as observing the phenomenon of interest (Bryman, 2004; Wolcott, 2002). A participant- observer is semi-involved when the need arises and functions as an observer most of the time, while a total observer observes without participation. An observer becomes a total participant where he/she participates fully in what is happening; a position most anthropologists adopt. Observing young inexperienced first time mothers learning to cope with a new role demanding application of new skills can be challenging.

- The health visitor as a clinician cannot avoid part participation. It would be inhuman to watch a young woman struggle to make a baby latch on flat nipples or watch her weep because her breasts are too full and painful without assisting. There are times when a health visitor can stand back and become a total observer especially when a woman performs self-care activities or other motherhood tasks efficiently (Bryman, 2004).

- Observations enable assessment of the knowledge deficit in the woman as she performs self-care and baby-care tasks. The health visitor will then note the identified knowledge gaps and use them in client education.

- Observation of the state of the woman's body post delivery reveals such anomalies like anaemia and oedema which the midwife should be able to manage immediately.

- Observations of the state of the woman's health should include the examination of the perineal area, Caesarean wounds, and the state of the breasts. Abnormal findings must be made and recorded.

- Women must be observed as they perform major tasks expected of them during the post natal period such as applying the baby to the breast for breast- feeding.

Ethical issues related to the use of observation must be observed (Wolcott,2002). Where the postnatal visits are two pronged, that is to provide care as well as collect essential data for improvement of care, women should consent to collection of information and they can consent to the recording of information and using it for improving care. Even where women know they are being observed they can respond freely to questions if the observer needs clarification of activities women engage in. Overt data that is data collected with the participants' knowledge can be collected and used in care interventions. The health visitor will notice that the interviewing and observations do not seem to worry women or alter the women's behaviours. Women are anxiously grappling with new roles and acquisition of skills expected of them and trying to meet the phase specific demands of the postnatal period. The women are addressing real life situations and going through a specific real life experience of the puerperium; they are only too happy to have a clinician watching them and providing advice.

Physical Examination

Postnatal examination is examination of the whole person, a full health assessment, to exclude minor and major physical, and mental problems that are likely to interfere with the health of the client and that of her infant.

- **A** home visit should include examination of the woman and baby after in-depth interviews.
- Being around the woman and getting an opportunity to examine the woman enables, assessment of her needs which enables provision of relevant health information as the woman is examined. Specific self -care skills and baby care skills should be imparted according to each woman's needs.
- It is advisable to examine the mother first.
- Discuss relevant topics like family planning and preparation for going back to work for the professional woman, and any topics of interest according to the client's need or the observations made.
- Observe the skills of baby care and discuss baby care he new mother. It is important to include the spouse or any other person such as mother, or grandmother who are likely to influence the young mother.
- Involvement of significant support person ensures that the young women have support in new skills and knowledge provided for by health personnel. Involvement of source of support in client education reduces conflict in self-care and baby care skills.
- Women and their source of support should be exposed to as much information as possible to reduce conflict and imposition of ineffective cultural postnatal practices (Wang et al., 2008; Helman, 2001).
- Each woman should have access to a leaflet on baby care skills or the baby milestones booklet as well as the booklets on self care and shaping up post delivery.

- Women and their sources of support should be given adequate time to express their fears and worries. A postnatal visit is as short or long as the individual woman requires help.

Baby Care

Primiparous clients require more time with the health visitor than other clients. It is not possible to equip a new mother with all the skills she requires during one visit. Simple postnatal problems like fixing baby to the breast, relieving breast engorgement may seem quite big to a young inexperienced first time mother. A home visit by health personnel provides solutions for small but 'big problems' to primiparous mothers, reassures them that they are applying the correct skills and enables them to develop confidence in self-care and baby care skills.

- On the first visit it is imperative to examine the baby from head to toe to pick out any abnormalities that may have been missed in hospital or that may have developed since leaving hospital (Morley,1979) .

- All reflexes must be tested.

- As the examination is going on, the mother can be advised on any issues that may arise as a result of the findings of the examination such as prevention of dehydration and signs of dehydration, care of the hair, heat rash, nappy rash, cleaning the umbilical stump and other skills (WHO,1998).

- The best way for a health visitor to assess skills in baby care is to suggest that the mother performs skills on the baby while the health visitor watches and advises. It is advisable that the health visitor observe the baby feeding in order to advise and respond to questions.

- On subsequent visits, the health visitor may want to reinforce on skills previously imparted as well as attend to specific requests from the client.

- Most baby care skills can be discussed and demonstrated in front of the new mother's source of support such as relative or hired domestic helpers. The working woman who plans to go back to work after a short while will welcome this approach.

- Whenever spouses are available they should be invited to participate in all activities during the visit. Involvement of spouses makes spouses aware of important issues in their families' health and makes them active participants in the care of their families.

Clients have their preferences; they should be consulted to participate in decision making and consent on any approach to their care before it is implemented (Liley,2001).

- The subsequent visit should be planned and a date and time comfortable for the client should be agreed upon.
- Women should be alerted of life-threatening conditions in the postnatal period and should know how to contact the nearest source of help. Each woman should have contact details of sources of help such as the health visitor, the hospital, the doctor and the ambulance.

A Post Natal Care Plan

After a thorough examination of the mother and the baby, the midwife and client plan the care of the client. A care plan has to be drawn in which manageable activities to be accomplished in one day are included. The care plan should be reviewed at every visit as mother's needs assessment is done. The midwife provides an advance organiser, which indicates how often she may be able to be with the mother, and the objectives of the visits based on the care plan.

In most care plans, there are five distinct activities namely, **assessing, planning, intervention, monitoring and evaluation.** In post-natal care, these phases are closely knit and sometimes interlinked that the distinction may not stand out. Every time the midwife visits the client, these skills are brought into play. It is important that the client is informed of any changes in the care plan, interventions and the need for referral to other members of the care team. The five activities repeated continuously during the course of care at specified intervals according to the client's condition. A day-to-day assessment enables monitoring of the client's state of health as well as observation for mastery of skills especially in primiparous clients.

References

1. Adler, P.A. and Adler, P. (1998). Observational techniques. In: Denzin, N.K. and Lincoln, Y.S. *Collecting and Interpreting Qualitative Materials*. Thousand Oaks, London, New Delhi: Sage Publications

2. Angrosino, M.V. and Mays de Perez, K.A. (2000). Rethinking Observation. From Method to Context. In: Denzin, N.K. and Lincoln, Y.S. *Handbook of Qualitative Research*. Thousand

Oaks, CA: Sage Publications.Bryman, A. (2004). *Social Research Methods*. Oxford: Oxford University Press.

3. Ellis, C. (1995). Doctor-Patient Relationship. *S.A. Family Practice*. 3, pp. 187-191.

4. Helman, C.G. (2001). *Culture, Health and Illness*. 4th ed. London: Arnold-Hodder.

5. Heron, J. (2001). *Helping the client. A Creative Guide*. 5th ed. Thousand Oaks, CA: Sage Publications.

6. Hope, T., Savulescu, J. and Hendrick, J. (2004). *Medical Ethics and Law*. Edinburgh: Churchill Livingstone.

7. Leininger, M.M. and McFarland, M.R. (2006). *Culture Care Diversity and Universality. A Worldwide Nursing Theory*. 2nd ed. London: Jones & Bartlett Publishers.

8. Ley, P. (1990). *Communicating with Patients*. London: Chapman and Hall

9. Liley, R., Lambden, P. and Newdick, C. (2001). *Understanding the Human Rights Act*. Abingdon: Radcliffe Medical Press Ltd.

10. Lloyd, M. and Bor, R. (2003). *Communication skills for Medicine*. Edinburgh: Churchill Livingstone Morley,D. Paediatric Priorities in the Developing World. Butterworths. 1979

11. Newell,R. Interviewing Skills for Nurses and other health care professionals.A structured approach.Routlegde,1994.

12. Polit, D.F;Hungler,B.P,Essentials of Nursing Research.Methods,Appraisal and Utilization. J.B. Lippincott Company.1993.Philadelphia

13. Richens,Y. Implementing the NICE guideline on postnatal care. The British Journal of Midwifery,2007,6(7) 412-417

14. Seedhouse, D. and Lovett, L. (1992). *Practical Medical Ethics*. Chichester: John Wiley and Sons.

15. Tenant, J.A. and Butler, M.S. (2007). Helping Women: the use of Heron's framework in Midwifery Practice. *British Journal of Midwifery*. 15(7), pp. 425-428.

16. Timmermans, D.R.M., Ockhuysen-Verney, C.F. and Henneman, L. (2005). Presenting health risk information in different formats: The effects on participants'cognitive and emotional evaluation and decisions. *Patient Education and Counselling*. 73(3), pp. 443-447.

17. UNFPA. (2006). *Maternal Mortality Update: Expectation and Delivery: Investing in Midwives and others with midwifery skills*. New York: United Nations Population Fund.

18. Wang, X., Wang, Y., Zanzhou, S., Wang, J. and Wang, J. (2008). A population based survey of women's traditional postpartum behaviours in Northern China. *Midwifery*. 24(2), pp. 238-245.

19. WHO. (1998). *Postpartum care of the mother and the newborn: a practical guide*. Geneva: World Health Organization.

20. Wimpenny, P. and Gass, J. (2000). Interviewing in Phenomenology and Grounded Theory: Is there a difference? *Journal of Advanced Nursing*. 31(6), pp. 1458-1492.

21. Ziervogel, C.F., Ahmed, N., Flisher, A.J. and Robertson, B.A. (1997). Alcohol misuse in South African male adolescents: A qualitative investigation. *International Quarterly of Community Health Education*. 17(1), pp. 25-41.

Chapter 4

THE PROCESS OF RECOVERY

The first week post delivery is a crucial period during which women who have just delivered babies take up their new roles as mothers. It is important that women are assisted to ease into these roles with evidence based support by competent health personnel. Becoming a mother is a life changing experience that gives a young woman a new position in society as a parent as well as increasing a woman's responsibilities of self-care, care of the newborn and care of the family. In some cultures having a baby enables participation and involvement in societal and cultural events as the woman may now be considered as an adult by virtue of being a mother (Mbizvo et al., 1993).

Early discharge from hospital post delivery is to encourage early ambulation and prevent complications such as infections and thrombo-embolic complications that a longer stay in hospital might result in. Early discharge home promotes confidence and an initiative to cope as best as possible with the situation a woman is faced with at the particular time. Professional support is especially essential for first time mothers and women who are prone to postnatal complications such as grand-multiparous women, and women who have had pregnancy and delivery complications.

Without professional support, a first time mother may be overwhelmed with new responsibilities of a baby and the bodily changes she may be experiencing. It is critical that a new mother quickly develops and applies appropriate self-care skills that address the physiological changes of her body she is currently experiencing (Orem, 1985).

Ideally women should be closely monitored post delivery and have on the average two visits at home after delivery from health professionals and should have up to five consecutive visits depending on their need (Hunter, 2008).

In many countries in Africa, there are no specific plans made in advance by health professionals to prepare the women for going home and there are no plans to offer the women professional support at home. Women are advised to visit the nearest health facilities should they need help. Review with health institutions after ten days and six weeks exposes many lives to postnatal complications and loss of lives during the time women are in their communities. If women's and newborn lives are to be saved, plans must be made as part of the health care delivery, to monitor women throughout the postnatal period from the third day after women leave health institutions.

Transformation

Becoming a mother is a process that transforms a young woman. Several changes take place within a short space of time challenging a woman to quickly manage all the demands such as change in the body function, body shape, sometimes physical scars, refocusing of feelings, increased responsibilities and high societal expectations.

The first week post delivery captures some of the new mother's dilemmas, emotions and needs at their peak. The woman is recovering from the effects of pregnancy and labour and awakening to an unusual almost shocking reality that she is no longer the same. Her body has undergone tremendous changes during pregnancy. She has undergone a shocking experience of labour and the experience has left her different in many ways. The woman is facing a new reality of the new person that she has become, a mother. She is likely to experience unexpected events within this new phase of life that may impact on her physical and mental well being. The first week post delivery is a crucial period in which professional support should be available for the new mother.

Recuperation

Quick recovery is desirable so that the woman returns to the normal female pre-pregnant cycle once more. There are practices in each community post delivery concerned with completion of the full cycle of femininity. Mature women in communities are concerned with quick healing and recovery of the women post delivery and that the woman gains strength and has restoration of good health so that she can take control of her new responsibility.

Elderly women in a family of a new mother, almost always keep a close eye on the new mother supervising and monitoring activities of the new mothers around self and the newborn baby using the limited resources and limited knowledge that they have. Practices and beliefs of a particular culture maybe similar irrespective of where they live, be it in the in the affluent suburbs or in peri-urban areas or in remote rural communities.

Women of the same cultures tend to share common knowledge and usually have in place a cultural 'routine' management of the normal puerperium. There can be rituals that young women have to follow supervised and enforced by elderly women in their families, and these are believed to enhance recovery and quick return to normalcy, but they may not all be safe and positively promoting good health. It is important that a health visitor familiarises herself with the client's cultural practices in order to offer safe but acceptable support without breaching the cultural norms of the respective community (Leinienger & MacFarland,2006).

Preserving Womanhood

In the postnatal period, young women tend to lean heavily on their pillars of support, the mature women in their families who have experience of child birth and this is more so in the absence of a credible source of information and support. Leaning on the mature and experienced women for support is a natural form of learning where the inexperienced learn through observation and trial and error under supervision until the young women are considered able to perform tasks and able to stand on their own. This way of learning appears to be a form of induction into roles, a process of growing up and maturing progressively into the phase of 'womanhood'. The young women are guided through advice and learning through living the experience during this crucial period. In one research, one young woman disclosed the advice she received from her grandmother. She said her grandmother told her:

'Listen to the advice I give you. If you miss this opportunity to learn about womanhood, you may never get another opportunity. I will not be around forever.' (Murira, 2010).

This statement suggests that in the female culture, cultural knowledge, values and practices are handed down from one woman to another and from one generation to the next (Mtambirwa, 1984). It also suggests that primiparous women are targets of numerous forms of advice from the popular sector of relatives, in-laws, neighbours and friends. It is important that professional support is accessible to advise on safe practices and provide health promotion advice.

It has been reported that women often feel poorly prepared for the post natal period and long for evidence based information and support during this period (Sword & Watt, 2005; Moore & Coty 2006). Some researchers have reported that poor staff attitudes and poor communication skills which may be prevalent in the postnatal period prevent prompt reporting of health problems and meeting women's felt needs (Brown et al., 2006). It is important that health personnel are familiar with the messages that are passed onto young mothers in communities to enable them to plan for provision of effective, relevant, client education and advice.

The community elderly women advisors may find difficulty in not only explaining but managing the unusual features occurring in the young women post delivery. It is therefore important that health personnel are at hand and accessible during the postnatal period to fill in the knowledge gaps and provide evidence based knowledge, skills and support. Some cultural beliefs and practices around a new mother are discussed in this section.

The Perineum

Some cultures like the Shona women's culture in Zimbabwe, believe that a 'well prepared perineum' before a woman goes into labour prevents bruising, ragged tears and the need for surgical cuts during labour. Preparation of the perineum before labour includes rituals to stretch the external opening of the vagina using varied objects. Primiparous women are however prone to bruising and tears of perineal muscle as their virgin muscles are stretched for the first time during the first delivery. The presence of perineal trauma in such a culture raises high levels of anxiety in the young women and their mentors as it is considered a shame in the respective culture. Perineal trauma and the surgical trauma (episiotomy) are seen as failure to follow traditional instructions and advice from the mature women during the last stages of pregnancy, the stage of preparation for labour. Both the young woman and her mentor are blamed by society for inflicting unnecessary injury on the perineum and for being responsible for causing vaginal opening distortion in case of trauma.

In the Shona women's culture there is a strong belief that if a woman had her perineum tempered with during labour, through perineal surgery or tears, the natural healing post delivery is interfered with and the shape of the vulva so distorted interfers with normal sexual activity post delivery. Episiotomy or perineal surgery is therefore abhorred, dreaded and despised in some cultures (Murira , 2010).

While some women may be able to deliver an average sized baby without sustaining a significant laceration or tear, some women may have very tight muscles which threaten to rapture immediately the pressure of the baby's head is on the perineum. Episiotomy is believed to ease the final stages of child birth, preventing injury to both the mother and baby especially where the head is large and likely to result in difficult delivery. Episiotomy is also done where delivery must be done quickly possible to save the infant.

Despite the positive benefits of an episiotomy, there is evidence that it is not a foolproof surgical procedure as some complications have been reported following an episiotomy such as possible increase in the likelihood of anal sphincter tearing, increased use of moderate to strong analgesia, postpartum haemorrhage, long term dyspareunia, incontinence of urine, incontinence of flatus and faeces and varied psychological impact (Macleod et al, 2008). Hidden internal lacerations may occur causing a steady loss of blood that may contribute to significant haemorrhage post delivery. Some of these complications can be prevented by thorough inspection of the lower segment of the uterus and vaginal vault immediately after the delivery of the placenta and prior to suturing and repair of damaged tissues.

For a long time, episiotomy has been accepted as a likely and sometimes inevitable procedure when delivering primiparous women vaginally, and is described as a 'routine procedure' with vaginal delivery in some first world societies (Murphy et al., 2008). There is however evidence that lacerations are associated with less blood loss compared with episiotomies and that cuts heal slowly compared to tears and bruises (Onah & Akani, 2004). There are suggestions that perineal trauma could be better managed by estimating the extent of trauma using an instrument called *peri-rule* (Metcalfe, 2004). The limitation of this instrument could be that it is only diagnostic and takes for granted professional skills like suturing and aseptic technique. In the abscence of wound management skills in a client, use of the instrument may not guarantee favourable perineal healing outcomes. A perineal management package that addresses professional skills, medical innovations and client education could be the answer to managing perineal trauma. Women who have sustained perineal trauma during childbirth have been found to be extremely uncomfortable, restless and in pain during the immediate puerperium and this has been reported to interfer with adopting comfortable positions that promote successful breastfeeding, severe pain on emptying bowels and during emptying of the bladder (Murira,2010).

In the Shona women's culture, the new mothers are exposed to many culturally accepted practices to 'heal the perineum' post delivery, especially where there are elderly members of the family to provide the much needed support during the immediate puerperium period. The Shona women's culture however is concerned with and has anxiety and urgency to contract the overstretched perineal muscles back to their pre-pregnant state and heal the perineal wounds as soon as possible with whatever means available to the mature women. Elderly women are believed to be the source of 'valuable' medicinal preparations that restore 'womanhood.'Many young women are advised and compelled by their women folk to wash the perineum three times a day using "herbal preparations" to 'contract the perineal muscles and heal the perineal wounds'. This practice was found to be so common that a health visitor sooner or later becomes familiar with the herbal preparation's typical astringent smell when freshly made and putrid smell when it is old and moldy (Murira,2010). The actual effects of cultural perineal treatments on the raw and tender perineum could be varied. It is possible that the practice is likely to expose women to the possibility of infection especially by the Tetanus bacteria considering that some 'treatment substances' are made from crushed fresh roots soaked in water. Research reports that community female elders load their advice with fear and that the young women are coerced into use of herbal treatments and engage in the practice out of fear of subsequent consequences as believed in their culture (Sutton,1982; Maddux & Rogers,1983) . The young women are urged through reassurances and instillation of fear messages to engage in the practices common in their culture and may be advised to tolerate unusual features of ill-health. Many of the young women who have had episiotomies express disappointment that their pre-delivery perineal preparation efforts are often in vain (Murira, 2010).

One belief supporting use of herbs is quoted below:

> 'The perineum is what is called a woman. It has to be toned back to shape with herbs while it is still tender to tighten the vaginal muscles. Loose vaginal muscles encourage wind to collect in the empty uterus resulting in a bulky abdomen.'(Murira,2010, interview extract)

An episiotomy is therefore regarded by some cultures as tempering with the *'woman'* since the perineum is *'womanhood'* itself. There are strong beliefs that a perineum that has been subjected to an episiotomy and extensive tears may never be the same again hence the anxiety to 'treat' the perineum and restore as much of the 'woman' as possible so that the woman recovers her perineal function as soon as possible. Muscle toning must therefore be done within a month or two before the young woman can return to her partner to become sexually active once more.

Health personnel should provide information and skills to tone up the perineal muscle through exercise as early as possible to encourage good blood flow and quick healing healing of the perineum to allow for sexual relationships to resume as early as possible.

Traditional use of plant pharmacology in reproductive health is described throughout the world (Ososkiet et al., 2002; Ticktin and Dalle, 2005; Martinez, 2008). These studies however are a result of interviews with traditional birth attendants and report on the objectives of the traditional birth attendants in prescribing the plant preparations. These researches reveal the beliefs of the birth attendants in the effectiveness of their prescriptions but there is no scientific evidence that supports effectiveness of these preparations in toning perineal muscles.

Many clients are unaware that body tissues recoil to their original structure and scars gradually resolve and completely disappear. Herbs ingested and inserted internally as remedies have a potential to cause renal disease, puerperal sepsis and cervical cancer. Professional advice and reassurance should be accessible to new mothers to convey evidence based information to anxious women and their mentors and dissuade women from practices whose effectiveness and benefits have not been proved. Third world countries especially in Africa have to invest in postnatal domiciliary care to prevent and reduce neonatal and maternal postnatal morbidity and mortality.

References

1. Hunter, L. (2008). Teenagers' experiences of postnatal care and breastfeeding. *British Journal of Midwifery*. 16(12), pp. 785-790.

2. Leininger, M.M. and McFarland, M.R. (2006). *Culture Care Diversity and Universality. A Worldwide Nursing Theory*. 2nd ed. London: Jones & Bartlett Publishers.

3. Macleod, M., Strachan, P., Bahl, R., Howarth, L., Goyder, K., Van de Venne, M. and Murphy D.J. (2008). A prospective cohort study of maternal and neonatal morbidity in relation to use of episiotomy at operative vaginal delivery. *BJOG: an International Journal of Obstetrics and Gynaecology*. 115(13), pp. 1688-1694.

4. Maddux, J.E. and Rogers, R.W. (1983). Protection Motivation and self-efficacy: a revised theory of fear appeals and attitude change. *Journal of Experimental Social Psychology*. 19, pp. 469-479.

5. Mbizvo,M.T; Fawcus,S; Lindmark,G et al., Maternal mortality in rural and urban Zimbabwe:social and reproductive factors in an incident case-referent study. *Social Science and Medicine*,1993; 36 (9):1197-205

6. Martinez, G.J. (2008). Traditional practices, beliefs and uses of medicinal plants in relation to maternal-baby health of Criollo woman in central Argentina. *Midwifery*. 24, pp. 490-502.

7. Metcalfe, A. (2004). Improving assessment of perineal tears: The Peri-Rule. *British Journal of Midwifery*. 12(10), pp. 618-220.

8. Mtambirwa, J. (1984). *Shona Pathology, Religion-Medical Practices and concepts of growth and development in relation to scientific medicine*. Harare: University of Zimbabwe.

9. Murphy, D.J., Macleod, M., Bahl, R., Goyder, K., Howarth, L. and Strachan, B. (2008). A randomised controlled trial of routine versus restrictive use of episiotomy at operative vaginal delivery: A multicentre pilot study. *BJOG*. 115(13), pp. 1695-1703.

10. Murira,N; Ashford,R; Sparrow,JCommunicating Sexual and Reproductive Health messages. Birmingham City University, Centre for Health and Social Care Research.(2010).

11. Onah, H.E; Akani, C.I. Rates and Predictors of Episiotomy in Nigerian Women. *Tropical Journal of Obstetrics and Gynaecology*, 2004; 21(1): 44-45

12. Orem, D.E.Nursing: Concepts of Practice 3rd ed. Mcgraw Hill, New York

13. Ososki, A.L., Lohr, P. and Reiff, M. (2002). Ethno-botanical literature survey of medicinal plants in the Dominican Republic used for women's health conditions. *Journal of Ethnopharmacology.* 79(3), pp. 285-298.

14. Sutton, S.R. *Fear Arousing Communications: a critical examination of theory and research.* In J.R. Eiser (ed). Social Psychology and Behavioural Medicine. London: Wiley, 1982: 307-37.

15. Ticktin, T. and Dalle, S.P. (2005). Medicinal plant use in the practice of midwifery in rural Honduras. *Journal of Ethnopharmacology.* 96(1-2), pp. 233-248.

Chapter 5

MORBIDITY POST DELIVERY

Many women suffer complications after leaving health institutions. Many health problems surface among the women in the first week of discharge from hospital and uninformed women may not realize how serious these problems are. Maternal morbidity is ill-health as a result of pregnancy related complications. Women may suffer physically and emotionally and their lives may be negatively altered permanently as a result of reproductive morbidity (Gessesewe &Melise,2002). Uncontrolled morbidity may lead to chronic ill-health or mortality.

Research has revealed that women's problems in the communities during the postnatal period are complex(Murira,2010) and that women are vulnerable during the post delivery period as they are exposed to high morbidity and mortality sometimes due to preventable causes such as haemorrhage, sepsis, anaemia, and eclampsia (Ariba et al., 2004; Nielson, 2003; Nwagha et al., 2004).

Before newly delivered mothers are sent home from health institutions, their age, experience and availability of support at home should be taken into consideration. In early discharge home, at the time the mothers leave hospital, some may not have recovered from the stress of labour. Complications may have not yet manifested. If young women are sent home within twenty-four hours post delivery without advice or support from health personnel, they have no choice but to depend on the knowledge and skills there is in the community in managing emerging health problems. Community based care skills may not always be effective practices and some may expose women to postnatal risks. Research has revealed that this approach is only for the survivors strong enough to find their way to these institutions and who can benefit from the services (Murira, 2001;Mbizvo, 1993)

Major causes of morbidity in the postnatal period are discussed.

Pain Post Delivery

Pain is an individual's response to sensitive and unpleasant physiological stimuli. It is the body's way to signal danger and discomfort. Pain intensity is thought to be influenced by the meaning of pain to the sufferer, the experience of pain, the expectations, the attitudes and beliefs and its expected duration (Williamson and Hoggart (2004). Primiparous women with no experience of previous child birth and may not know what to expect feel genuine pain that is not influenced by beliefs or attitudes or based on previous experience.

Research of pain post delivery revealed that pain perception seemed to increase with parity suggesting that primiparous women's perceptions were probably underplayed by lack of experience (Jangsten, 2005).

Origins of Post delivery pain :

- Bruised, and lacerated birth canal
- Stretched and bruised adenaxae
- After pains of labour due to the uterine contraction as involution occurs
- Post-surgical wound pain (Macleod et al., 2008).

Post delivery pain interferes with sleep, breastfeeding, emptying bowels and bladder and the general well being of the woman. Pain may cause hallucinations, restlessness and a rise in temperature. Clients choose to have their babies in health institutions so that the process of childbirth is made as comfortable as possible and relief of pain contributes immensely to this comfort. The attitude of many people including some health personnel is that the pain of childbirth should be tolerable and assume that it should go away soon after the delivery of the baby. Women have reported considerable pain and discomfort that health personnel have tended to take little notice of after delivery (Murira et al., 2003). Pain is more severe in women who deliver surgically, and those who have had assisted deliveries. Women report post delivery pain of varied severity as described below:

'The pain *was as severe as the pain of labour,*

'*The pain disturbed my sleep at night'*

'*It felt very uncomfortable; my partner had to buy analgesics for me from the local pharmacy'*

'*I went to see the local GP. I couldn't imagine another night in such pain'*

"*I just felt intense heat, sweated and shivered at the same time."*

"*It felt like labour pain had come back. The pain made me sleepless."*

'*I was in such pain the last two days. It made me restlessness and unable to find a comfortable enough position to sit or lye in"* (Murira,2010).

From the statements above, it is clear that pain threshold varies from one individual woman to another. What one post-natal mother may consider mild and tolerable pain may be considered severe pain by another. Women's' requests for pain relief should be taken seriously and potent analgesics should be given initially in the first forty-eight hours, followed by mild analgesics, as the client feels more comfortable. Clients have to be individualized in care to meet their needs satisfactorily. Health personnel must be empathetic to clients to prevent unnecessary discomfort post delivery.

Headache

Women have reported headaches post delivery. The most common cause of headache post delivery has been found to be high blood pressure (Murira,2010). New cases of high blood pressure may suddenly emerge post delivery in women who may not have had high blood pressure before. Any complaints of headache post delivery must be thoroughly investigated. Every woman must have her blood pressure checked on each home visit.

Headaches post- natally, may be due to lack of sleep because of the baby's demands, and anxiety about the added responsibility. Many primiparous women may need advice to plan their time and find time to rest. A new mother must try to sleep when the baby sleeps so that when the baby is awake and active the mother is also alert. There is need for postnatal domiciliary support to enable diagnosis of pain and efficient management of pain.

Hypertension

Hypertension is ranked as the second most common health problem postnatal mothers suffer from. Women, who may have not suffered from high blood pressure previously, or with the last pregnancy, may be found to be hypertensive post delivery. Many women may not be aware what could be making them feel unwell. Women may not be familiar with the symptoms of high blood pressure and may not know the risk associated with high blood pressure.

Postnatal mothers' lack of knowledge of hypertension is reflected in the statements below.

'My feet are swollen, I cannot wear shoes. I have no idea what it is.'

'I have a severe headache, dizziness, and intense heat in my chest. I think the headache is because I have not slept well for the past two nights.'

'I have a headache that won't go away even after a rest or taking paracetamol.

'I feel dizzy I do not know why, perhaps I am tired. Isn't it that's what happens after delivery'(Murira,2010).

Murira, (2010), found that eclampsia was least understood by women who associated it with *attacks by strong evil spells from jealous enemies*. Eclampsia is a complication of pre-eclampsia and is characterized by convulsions. This is a serious complication that may result in renal failure, cerebral oedema and loss of life (Friedlander, 2008; Peters, 2008). High incidence of eclampsia in the postnatal period has been reported by researchers in other African communities (Obiechina and Udigwe (2004).

Researchers report that certain cultures regard negative health outcomes as omens or punishments for wrong doing while other cultures look for someone to blame for every misfortune and ill health in their lives (Lupton, 1999). In a study of community perception of the causes of maternal mortality, Umoiyoho and Abbasiattai (2005) report that the community they studied associated maternal death with spiritual attacks from enemies and punishment by gods for infidelity. This is suggesting that causes of ill health and mortality among indigenous Africans are believed to be extraneous and mysterious and are associated with enmity and wrong doing. This suggests that client education among African communities and especially among women should address beliefs and superstition as well as providing scientific explanations to obstetric complications.

Post natal obstetric complications including eclampsia are reported to be among the major causes of morbidity and mortality among women of the reproductive age group in Cambodia (Yanagisawa & Wakai ,2008). Research among 11-12 year olds and 17-18 year old non-pregnant females in India identified a spurt of high blood pressure among the adolescents suggesting that hypertensive disease is likely to occur among primiparous women (Saha et al., 2008).

The prevalence of high blood pressure among primiparous women in the post delivery period emphasizes the importance of empowering women with relevant information that enables them to recognize the symptoms of hypertension early to enable them to make informed decisions to seek health care services promptly. A maternal mortality survey in Zimbabwe revealed that 15.7% of maternal deaths were due to hypertension in pregnancy and eclampsia (Munjanja et al., 2007). The presence of post natal complications minor or major suggests that there is a need for professional monitoring of women post delivery to exclude the complications and to support women with relevant education and information to improve their self-care skills.

Wound Complications

Not all women are competent to deal with postnatal complications especially something unusual, such as wound complications arising unexpectedly.

Critical Incident 2

One woman was found by a health visitor during a post natal visit lying on a bed with half of her bowels out of the abdominal wall. Pus flowed out of the open wound. She was pyrexial and almost in shock. She told the health visitor:

"The wound opened as I got out of bed. The wound has been oozing small amounts of pus from the first day I came from hospital. I use tissue paper to wipe off the discharge. I thought it would heal shortly. I was going to wait until my husband comes back from work for him to decide what we can do. " (Murira,2010).

Poor wound healing and poor wound management has been observed in the postnatal period and women have been observed to use anything they can get hold of from salt, petroleum jelly, tissue paper and cloth to manage raw suture lines and oozing wounds, increasing the likelihood of infection and morbidity (Murira,2010). Researchers have reported that women do not have adequate information about caesarean delivery and what to expect thereafter (Horey et al., 2004). The desperate wound management efforts suggest a pressing need for a professional support system for women during the postnatal period. Lack of decision making powers among the women population, the lack of post natal support, the inability to freely access health services and the non-existent means to communicate with the nearest health facilities in emergencies exposes women in the third world to postnatal morbidity.

Perineal Sepsis

Cases of perineal sepsis, offensive vaginal discharge, and broken down perineal wounds have been observed among young women (Murira ,2010). The underlying cause of these post natal problems may not be obvious. There are possibilities that the cultural management of the perineum, the herbal washes, and the surgical technique especially the suturing and underlying conditions such as HIV and diabetes, may slow down wound healing.

Cultural perineal healing practices could be an indication of an unmet need for information on perineal care in women, the process of involution, wound healing and tissue repair. Some cultural practices potentially exposure the young women to puerperal sepsis especially bacterial and fungal infections. It is important that the young women have access to information on perineal care. Cultural perineal healing practices suggest that women need effective information, a gap that should be filled in by effective antenatal education throughout pregnancy as well as post delivery education support (Onah & Akani, 2004).

Symphyseal Bone Dysfunction

If a woman fails to walk the next morning after a vaginal delivery and has severe pain on the pubic area, the most likely cause is symphyseal bone dysfunction as related by one woman:

"My legs just won't move; I have excruciating pain in my hips. I have to crawl to the toilet. It is not easy. I cannot straighten my legs. It is like I'm breaking my bones below my waist." I thought the pain would go away soon and that I would be able to walk again soon" (Murira ,2010)

Symphyseal bone pain may be felt during delivery when the joint separation occurs and can be felt while a woman is still in hospital but there has to be thorough and proper examination including xrays to assess and diagnose the magnitude of the problem. Without professional advice and support, a woman may not perceive the likely source of the pain and the severity of the problem. If women receive information on likely labour complications during the antenatal period just around 36weeks of gestation the information could assist them in risk awareness and risk identification during and immediately after labour.

The diagnosis of symphyseal bone dysfunction in the first week post delivery justifies the need for a postnatal support system for women to make prompt diagnosis to alleviate pain and reduce morbidity among women affected.

Bladder complications

Bladder complications may develop in some women within the first week at home after delivery but may be at a loss as to what to do to care for themselves. One woman related:

> 'I keep on going to the toilet and the urine burns. I felt like this in pregnancy and I thought perhaps it was part of the feeling one gets in pregnancy. I am surprised these symptoms have re-surfaced after delivery.' (Murira, 2010)

Women who have had a second degree perineal tear are likely to have hesitancy to empty the bladder due to pain and bruising of the perineal muscles. Some women may fail to pass urine resulting in a full bladder and a distended abdomen. Women are further exposed to morbidity by delays to seek health care, adopting a *'wait and see"* attitude especially if they lack resources to seek transport and where there is 'fee for service' health care policies as one woman reported:

> 'My abdomen is sore. I won't drink any more fluids because the abdominal pain is getting worse. I have not passed urine since yesterday morning. I can't possibly sit down to pass urine. I have so much pain down below. I can't call an ambulance because we cannot afford it. I just have to wait and see, maybe I will manage to pass urine.' (Murira, 2010).

A woman with poor control of the bladder after a difficult assisted delivery had this to say:

> 'I keep on wetting myself when I laugh and sometimes I just find myself wet. It is very embarrassing. I have to stay in my room; I can't join the rest of the family in case I wet myself.'

Dysuria is associated with poor asceptic technique during labour and perineal repair, too many vaginal examinations, and inadequate treatment of urinary tract infection in pregnancy. Bladder problems post vaginal delivery in particular retention of urine, are associated with difficult labour in primiparous women, and prolonged first and second stages of labour. Bladder problems are also associated with epidural anaesthesia and instrumental delivery, as well as birth canal and perineal trauma (Teo et.al.,2007). Urine retention post delivery is associated with damage to nerves and hypotonic pelvic musculature (Glavind, 2004). Bladder problems especially the lack of control of the bladder, affect women psychologically temporarily or permanently. Women so affected may resort to self-isolation because of the embarrassment of the urine leakage and the smell of urine on the person and wherever they sit. Bladder control problems usually respond to Kegel or pelvic floor muscle exercises post delivery.

Women need support from health professionals to master these exercises during pregnancy and after delivery to achieve effective control of the bladder. Provision of information, skills, continuous support and encouragement from antenatal period through to the post natal period by health personnel, should help women to experience less bladder complications, enable them to identify bladder complications early and promptly seek attention. Provision of health information to women and communities reduces morbidity and saves women's lives.

Haemorrhoids

The discomfort of haemorrhoids postnatally is reported by researchers (Abramowitz& Batallan, 2003). During late pregnancy, the effect of progesterone on smooth muscles affects the tone of the pelvic floor and perineal muscles. The weight of the gravid uterus causes pressure on these muscles and blood vessels sag and swell. The swollen blood vessels may rapture during a bowel motion causing bleeding during and after a bowel motion. These painful, sagging and sometimes bleeding blood vessels are called haemorrhoids.

During labour the pressure of the baby on the bowel as the baby pushes his way out causes further sagging of the blood vessels around the bowel opening and the whole perineal area. After delivery the loose blood vessels may continue to cause pain during bowel movements and after bowel movements. Some blood vessels may burst out and bleed with each bowel movement. Swollen and bleeding haemorrhoids distress women post delivery as one woman stated:

'It is difficult to sit after a bowel motion. I have to lye on my side, but even then I am in a lot of pain.'

Haemorrhoids distress women and many amateur cultural attempts to treat haemorrhoids have been observed. Some herbal treatments have been observed to excoriate the perineum and cause severe puerperal sepsis.

Women should be advised to keep the perineal area clean to prevent infection of the rectal area which may result in peri-anal abscesses. Haemorrhoids should disappear by the end of two to three weeks post delivery; but should they persist, a woman should be advised to see a GP for further management.

The presence of post delivery complications among women in the first week post delivery confirm that the postnatal period is fraught with health problems and that women require professional attention and support post delivery. Postnatal professional support is not available; women have been reported to rely on cultural herbal 'treatments' to address postnatal complications. Without professional supervision post delivery, women are exposed to high levels of morbidity and possible mortality.

A study on utilization of postnatal care services in one district in Zimbabwe failed to account for a tenth of the would be users of the service (Hove et al, 1999). It is possible that women fail to turn up at clinics for postnatal services because of varying degrees of postnatal complications. It is possible that some may have lost their lives. Women may not value a service being offered after they have survived the most critical part of the post natal period in which they most needed help.

Risk Perception

Lack of urgency to seek health care services is a behaviour that can be caused by several factors. Women may have no knowledge of the postnatal complications and may have no idea of the implications of the postnatal events on their health. Where women have visible discomfort, women may find it expensive to seek further health care services after the delivery of the baby.

There may be lack of awareness of the value of health care services within the environment in which the woman lives. The community may have high values of their own cultural management of childbirth and care of the new mother.

Culture helps one to understand risk in a particular cultural context and this is a communal notion of risk and not an individualistic view. Culture determines which risks are high risks worth worrying about (Lupton, 1999).

Where women do not get professional advice as an alternative to cultural teaching, women may rely on their tradition and culture and may not have the ability to identify risks to their health. In the absence of scientific evidence based information, clients' awareness of risk can only be understood from a socio-cultural point of view. A socio-cultural view of risk is unlikely to have similar meanings of the severity of risk and pay the risk the urgency the risk deserves. Risk may not be interpreted and seen from the health professional's perspective. The clients are unlikely to adopt appropriate behaviours as expected by health personnel or apply effective self-care skills where they do not realize that their lives are at risk. Without professional advice, women practise what comes naturally to them, what they know, what is easy and affordable to them and what is supported by the society in which they live.

Cultural diversity and postnatal behaviours

Culture is a particular group of people's beliefs, norms, values, rules of behaviour, and lifestyle practices, system of symbols with shared values, meanings and behavioural norms that are learned and shared and guide decisions and actions in a patterned manner (Leininger & McFarland,2006).Culture is humane –oriented; members of a culture spend time together, extend empathy and love and share information to solve their problems (House et al, 2004). Culture is the broadest, most comprehensive, holistic, and universal feature of human beings (Kavanagh & Kennedy (1992; Leininger, 2007). Cultural differences emerge where ways of life, values, beliefs, ideals and practices are concerned and depend on the degree of heterogeneity of those interacting.

Every culture has its own beliefs and practices around pregnancy, labour and childbirth hence the need for health personnel to be familiar with their clients' culture (Paradice, 2002; Greene, 2007). Although childbirth is a universal experience among women, and each woman's childbirth experience is unique and health personnel should be cognisant of this unique experience in each client. Health care involves meeting and interacting with people from diverse cultures, trying to understand, inform, advise and influence, counsel and console them (Tanvantanakul et al.,2006). Activities of health personnel when dealing with their clients call for an understanding of the clients culture (Kavanagh &Kennedy,1992).

Health care is embedded in culture and cultures expect to receive meaningful health care that respects their cultural values and ways of life as a human right (Leininger &

MacFarland, (2006). Understanding women's culture in reproductive health enables untapped and essential knowledge to reproductive health care to be brought to light to enrich reproductive health care practice. Culture plays a major role in a woman's beliefs, values and practices and how she prepares for the childbirth experience.

Understanding Clients' Culture

Culturally based reproductive health care practice should lead to understanding women better and should be capitalised on to increase risk perception among women as health personnel and women exchange information in discussions. Midwives have the opportunity to increase health promoting information in women and influence change of attitudes through the incorporation of the cultural aspect of care into the care of women. A culturally competent midwife can support and promote education and also advocate for women to meet their specific cultural needs in pregnancy, childbirth and post delivery (Greene, 2007). Understanding the cultures of women enables midwives to respect their clients' culture and to offer care that does not offend their clients (Thomson, 1997).

Understanding clients' culture enables cultural negotiation and cultural accommodation so that health personnel and clients work towards similar goals. Accepting and respecting the differences between and among people is part of inter-personal relationships and helps to understand the client's perspective and understanding the client's needs. Improved health personnel-client communication therefore enables analysis and development of strategies for intervention to improve clients' health (Kavanagh & Kennedy, 1992). The challenges for establishing effective interventions that can challenge ineffective and potentially dangerous cultural practices are greater and require objectivity, determination, a critical mind especially where health personnel and clients come from similar cultures. Culturally based knowledge is needed in such interventions to meet the needs of the people and to provide culturally accepted and healing care while taking care not to cause conflict with the people's culture (Leininger, 2007). Culture care should enable discovery of similarities and differences in health care practice, values, beliefs and practices between health professionals and the clients they serve.

Healthcare clients have *emic* knowledge which comes directly from their culture that is, from their beliefs, values and practices in their indigenous cultural contexts; while *etic* knowledge comes from health personnel's views of care values (Leininger (2007). Both emic and etic care values are essential to devise congruent and acceptable care which promotes the client's well-being, enables prevention of ill- health by creating culturally accepted awareness of ill health, shortens the client's recovery time from ill health, and reduces the client's cost of health care. Understanding clients' culture reduces cultural conflicts between health personnel and their clients and the despondency that can emerge. Cultural understanding therefore enables sustenance of culturally accepted quality reproductive health care at the same time improving the care by blending what the client already knows with new information (Leininger & McFarland, 2006; Leininger, 2007).

Balancing different Cultures

Balancing cultural differences consists of three health care actions namely culture care preservation or maintenance, culture care accommodation, and culture care repatterning or restructuring which form the guidelines to use culturally based values beliefs and practices with active participation of health care clients (Leininger & McFarland, 2006). The most universal and dominant construct of cultural care has been identified as that of respect for and about cultures (Leininger, 2007). The proponents of the culture care paradigm suggest that culture care enables health personnel to value and respect cultural differences helps health personnel to deal with their biases and misconceptions about different cultures. Cultural congruence has therefore the power to promote wellness and make professional health services fit into the clients' way of life (Leininger, 2007).

Competence in a people's culture

Cultural competence is based on a strong foundation of knowledge about a particular culture(s). It is important that health personnel who are in contact with women from various cultural orientations develop cultural competence of the women they are looking after. Cultural competence creates awareness of the impact of cultural, the socio-economic factors and their influence on women's health. Cultural competence enables health personnel to use the appropriate language, observe acceptable norms, and help women access safe health care that responds to their health care needs while still observing their culturally acceptable birth practices.

The theory of culture care diversity and universality is useful in critically analyzing communication relationships of health personnel and their clients and how this relationship impacts on women's satisfaction with care and women's health in general(Leininger and

McFarland,2005). This critical analysis is essential for mapping out of strategies to make reproductive health care and practice blend with the women's culture in order to increase risk perception in women and reduce maternal morbidity and mortality.

Social cognitive models (Bandura, 1977, 1986) regard behaviour as emanating from cognitions commonly shared by society. Social cognition places value and concern of a person on their social world around them. The Theory of Reasoned Action reaffirms Bandura's theory by suggesting that behaviour unfolds within a context influenced by social norms and beliefs.

There are several external cues according to the Health Belief Model(Becker&Maimen, 1957), that are modifying factors to behaviours to include socio-cultural factors, the cultural explanation of a problem, and if the particular society appreciates one's circumstances and experiences as a problem. The age of the individual for instance is a major modifier of behaviour which can affect young women's decision- making powers as well as their self-care and baby care skills.

First time mothers and women who have never accessed scientific knowledge may not possess deep understanding of health in general let alone reproductive health issues. The elderly family members may see it as their responsibility to lead and control in the health care and behaviours of young women throughout the post natal period.

The general lack of basic knowledge of what constitutes "risk" in both the young women and their mentors, the absence of a back up health service in the form of a domiciliary postnatal service, and the non-existence of complementary leaflets and books to empower women with information may further expose women to morbidity in the postnatal period.

Reducing postnatal morbidity and mortality requires a women centred sexual and reproductive health policy that embraces many sectors. In many developing countries, women's health begins to take prominence when a woman falls pregnant and the pre-pregnancy stage is rarely given attention. Adolescent sexual health in schools should be standardised and specific to increase health consciousness in young people to prevent teenage pregnancies and early exposure of young people to sexual and reproductive morbidity (Reeves et al,2006). It has been reported that many sexually active adolescents in many parts of Africa lack information on sexual health (Biddlecom et al., 2007). An informed young population is likely to have an increased risk awareness and reduced incidence of adverse reproductive health incidents.

References

1. Abramowitz, A. and Batallan, A. (2003). Epidemiology of anal lesions (fissure and thrombosed external haemorrhoid) during pregnancy and postpartum. *Gynécologie, obstétrique & fertilité*. 31(6), pp. 546-549.

2. Ariba, A.J., Inem, A.V., Biersack, G., Aina, O.A., Ayankogbe, O.O. and Adetoro, O.O. (2004). Pattern of Obstetric Mortality in A Voluntary Agency Hospital in Abeokuta South West Nigeria. *Nigerian Medical Practitioner*. 45(5), pp. 83-90.

3. Bandura, A. (1977). *Social learning theory*. Englewood Cliffs, NJ: Prentice Hall.

4. Bandura, A. (1986). *Social foundations of thought and action*. Englewood Cliffs, NJ: Prentice Hall.

5. Becker, M.H. and Maiman, L.A. (1983). Models of health-related behaviour. In: Mechanic, D. *Handbook of Health, Health Care and the Health Professions*. New York: Free Press.

6. Biddlecom, A.E., Munthali, A., Singh, S. and Woog, V. (2007). Adolescents views of and preferences for sexual and reproductive health services in Burkina Faso, Ghana, Malawi and

   Uganda. *African Journal of Reproductive Health*. 11(3), pp. 99-100.

7. Friedlander, F. (2008). Pre-eclampsia, a high risk complication of pregnancy: the implications for antenatal, intra-partum and postnatal care. *MIDIRS Midwifery Digest*. l18(4), pp. 505-509.

8. Gessessew, A. and Melese, M.M. (2002). Ruptured uterus eight year retrospective analysis of

   causes and management outcome in Adigrat Hospital, Tigray Region, Ethiopia. *Ethiopian Journal of Health Development*. 16(3), pp. 241-245.

9. Glavind, K. (2004). Incidence and treatment of urinary retention postpartum. *International*

   Urogynecology Journal. 14(2), pp. 119-121.

10. Greene, M.J. (2007). Stategies for Incorporating Cultural Competence into Childbirth Education Curriculum. *Journal of Perinatal Education*. 16(2), pp. 33-37.

11. Horey, D., Weaver, J. and Russel, J. (2004). Information for pregnant women about caesarean birth. *Cochrane Database of Systematic Reviews*. (1), CD003858.

12. House, R.J., Hanges, P.J., Javidan, M., Dorfman, P.W. and Gupta, V. (2004). *Culture,*

Leadership, and Organizations. London: Sage Publications.

13. Hove, I., Siziya, S. and Katito, C. (1999). Prevalence and associated factors for non-utilization of Post Natal Care Services: Population-Based Study in Kuwadzana Peri-Urban Area, Zvimba District of Mashonaland West Province, Zimbabwe. *Central African Journal of Medicine*. 50(6), pp. 39-45.

14. Jangsten, E., Strand, R., Gomez de Freitas, E., Hellström, A.L., Johansson, A. and Bergström, S. (2005). Women's perceptions of pain and discomfort after childbirth in Angola. *African Journal of Reproductive Health*. 9(3):148-158.

15. Kavanagh, K.H. and Kennedy, P.H. (1992). *Promoting cultural diversity: strategies for health care professionals*. Newbury Park, CA: Sage Publications.

16. Leininger, M.M. and McFarland, M.R. (2006). *Culture Care Diversity and Universality. A Worldwide Nursing Theory*. 2nd ed. London: Jones & Bartlett Publishers.

17. Leininger, M.M. (2007). Theoretical Questions and Concerns: Response from the Theory of

    Culture Care Diversity and Universality Perspective. *Nursing Science Quarterly*. 20(9), pp. 9-13.

18. Lupton, D. (1999). *RISK*. London and New York: Routledge.

19. Macleod, M., Strachan, P., Bahl, R., Howarth, L., Goyder, K., Van de Venne, M. and Murphy D.J. (2008). A prospective cohort study of maternal and neonatal morbidity in relation to use of episiotomy at operative vaginal delivery. *BJOG: an International Journal of Obstetrics and Gynaecology*. 115(13), pp. 1688-1694.

20. Mbizvo, M.T., Fawcus, S., Lindmark, G., Nyström, L. (1993). Maternal mortality in rural and

    urban Zimbabwe: social and reproductive factors in an incident case-referent study. *Social*

    Science and Medicine. 36(9), pp. 1197-11205.

21. Munjanja, S.P. (2007). *Maternal and Perinatal Mortality Study*. Zimbabwe: Ministry of Health and Child Welfare Zimbabwe.

22. Murira,N.(2013) Communicating Sexual and Reproductive Messages: In search of a model to increase risk perception among primiparous women.Birmingham City University.PhD Thesis.

23. Murira, N. (2006). *Pregnancy, Labour, Self-Care and Baby Care*. Maryland, USA: Publish

America.

24. Murira, N., Lützen, K., Lindmark, G. and Christensson K. (2003). Communication patterns

    between health personnel and their clients in an antenatal clinic in Zimbabwe. *Journal of*

    Women's Health. 24(2), pp. 83-92.

25. Nielson, J.P. (2003). *Interventions for treating placental abruption. Cochrane Database of*

    Systematic Reviews. (1), CD003247.

26. Nwagha, U.I., Okaro, J.M. and Nwagha, T.U. (2004). The third stage of labour - A Time Bomb. *Journal of College of Medicine.* 9(1), pp. 14-19.

27. Obiechina, N.J.A. and Udegbe, C.B. (2003). Maternal Mortality at St. Charles Borromeo Hospital, Onitsha: A Six Year Review. *Orient Journal of Medicine.* 15(2), pp. 26-30.

28. Onah, H.E. and Akani, C.I. (2004). Rates and Predictors of Episiotomy in Nigerian Women.

    Tropical Journal of Obstetrics and Gynaecology. 21(1), pp. 44-45.

29. Paradice, R. (2004). *Psychology for Midwives.* Trowbridge: Cromwell Press.

30. Peters, M. (2008). High Blood Pressure in Pregnancy. *Nursing for Women's Health.* 12(5), pp. 413-421.

31. Reeves, C., Whitaker, R., Parsonage, R.K., Robinson, C.A., Swale, K. and Bayley, L. (2006).

    Sexual Health Services and Education: Young people's experiences and preferences. *Health*

    Education. 65(4), pp. 368-379.

32. Saha, I., Paul, B. and Dasgupta, A. (2008). Short communication: Prevalence of hypertension

    and variation of blood pressure with age among adolescents in Chetla, India. *Tanzania Journal of Health Research.* 10(2), pp. 108-111.

33. Tanvatanakul, V., Amado, J. and Saowakontha, S. (2007). Management of communication

    channels for health information in the community. *Health Education Journal.* 66(2), pp. 173-

178.

34. Teo, R., Punter, J., Abrams, K., Mayne, C. and Tincello, D. (2007). Clinically overt postpartum urinary retention after vaginal delivery: a retrospective case-control study. International Urogynecology *Journal and Pelvic Floor Dysfunction.* 18(5), pp. 521-524.

35. Thomson, A. (1997). Learning from the community about barriers to health care. *Obstetrics and Gynaecology.* 87(1), pp. 140-141.

36. Umoiyoho, A.J., Abasiattai, A.N., Udoma, E.J. and Etuk, S.J. (2005). Community perception of the causes of maternal mortality among the the Annang of Nigeria's South-East coast. *Tropical Journal of Obstetrics and Gynaecology.* 22(2), pp. 189-192.

37. Williamson,A;Hoggart,B.(2005) Pain: a review of three commonly used pain rating scales.

    Journal of Clinical Nursing,14,pp798-804. Plackwell Publishing Ltd.

38. Yanagisawa, S. and Wakai, S. (2008). Professional healthcare use for life-threatening obstetric conditions. *Journal of Obstetrics and Gynaecology.* 28(7), pp. 713-719.

Chapter 6

SELF-CARE

Self-Care is the application of effective skills to manage physiological, developmental and individual's health needs. It is engagement in activities that maintain life as a response to a current demand be it situational, developmental or health related need.

The objectives of self-care are to :

- Cope with current situation and impending situation
- Maintain good health
- Improve one's quality of life and
- Prevent adverse events that compromise one's health

Self-care skills can be divided into three major categories namely;

- Universal or physiological self-care skills
- Developmental self-care skills
- Health deviation self-care skills(Orem,1985).

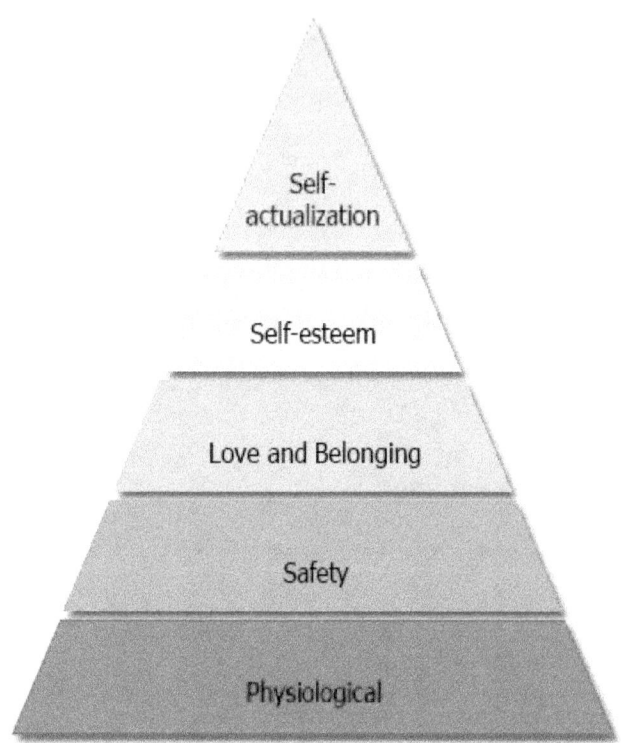

Fig. 6.1Maslow's Hierarchy of Human Needs (Maslow, 1954; 1971)

Maslow's hierarchy of human needs suggests that every human being seeks to fulfil a hierarchy of needs that enables her to survive and feel some satisfaction in life. The needs are illustrated in the above triangle and show the basic and initial needs at the bottom of the triangle. An individual aspires to achieve one level of need before aspiring for a higher level and is not satisfied until she attains the highest level of needs, the self actualisation.

Universal self -care needs

These are basic physiological needs that sustain life e.g.shelter, food, fresh air. Every individual needs these d4mand that one has self-care skills to survive and attain the requirements essential to survive. One engages in specific activity to ensure access to these needs. Universal self -care skills can be developed intuitively as a response to suit the environment and the prevailing circumstances (Orem, 1985). One has to look for food, prepare it to survive. One has to make some form of shelter or seek shelter to protect oneself against wind, rain, cold or heat. One must ensure that they are safe from danger . These needs are across gender, age or colour and physical boundaries; they apply to every human being.

Developmental self care needs arise along the life-line as one approaches a higher phase in the process of growing up. As a woman develops along the lifeline from a girl child, an

74

adolescent, a young woman and a mother, she is therefore expected to display phase specific skills expected of the specific stage she has reached along the life line. One has to be able to deal with the bodily needs as dictated by the phase of development and as expected by society. Ability to apply phase specific skills determines physiological maturity and enables society to determine and differentiate between normal physical development and maturity and subnormal development.

Developmental self -care needs therefore:

- Respond to factors affecting the growth cycle
- Enable adjustment to suit the requirements for a specific level of development such as the transition from a girl-child to adolescence and from an adolescent to a woman.
- Specific to meet the demands of each stage of development.
- Are learned behaviour learnt and refined through observation and practice from significant others, culture, and through socialization to regulate human functioning and development triggered by one's needs (Comely, 1994).
- Are life long behaviour adjusted to suit specific challenges that an individual meets along the life span.

Health deviation self-care needs

The health deviation self-care skills are subdivided into :

- Wholly compensatory skills,
- Partial compensatory skills and
- Supportive or educational self-care skills People apply their own self-care skills responding to the demands of illness, disease and emergency situations until they have reached the limit of their capabilities.
- People seek assistance from others when their self- care skills are exhausted. This is the point at which they are likely to be influenced by others around them (Comely, 1994).
- At this stage a person may seek therapeutic self- care offered by health professionals.

The roles of health professionals are:

- Supporting and strengthening the existing skills already in the client and

- Upgrading the care skills the client already has through communication and information giving,
- The **goal** of health personnel should be that of helping people meet their own self-care demands.
- Health personnel may assist their clients to perform those skills clients cannot perform and those skills are at three levels of health care.

Wholly compensatory health care

- Health personnel provide care that caters for the total inability of an individual to perform self-care activities.
- Care given to clients who are incapacitated by chronic illness or physical disability.
- This care for unconscious or semi-conscious clients following surgical procedures involving general anaesthesia, and in comatose clients.

Partial compensatory care

- Involves assisting the clients for partial inability to perform self-care activities.
- It is offered to clients in the process of recuperating from debilitating illness and after major surgery (Orem,1985) and also to clients adjusting to new situations and conditions that the client must learn to live with such as following delivery of a baby.
- It is best combined with the supportive/educational self-care skills.

The supportive/ Educative level of self-care

- Involves assisting clients in acquiring knowledge and skills that lead to informed decision-making and application of appropriate behaviours that support good health.
- It is accomplished through the use of health promotion.
- The health personnel's role at this level changes to be that of *an empowerer* and facilitator in acquisition of relevant information that improves a client's health (Jewell, 1994).
- The client is exposed to full information on her health in order to increase her confidence to participate in her self-care.
- The teaching role of the health care provider is greatly emphasized. Through the support, the client develops confidence in performing skills and taking responsibility for her own health

- It increases client's satisfaction in health care (Madnick, 1980; Ballard -Reisch, 1990).

Prerequisites of Effective self -care

- The client must have access to relevant information that continuously provides knowledge of strategies that promote quality health such as what constitutes healthy food, the health issues and behaviours that endanger an individual's life, what constitutes emergencies, what are the effective measures to respond to the emergencies and prevent loss of life and the ability to apply these measures to one's life.
- The client must be fully involved as a full participant in decision-making in matters concerning her care
- The client must enjoy continuous support from the health professional to give her confidence in her self-care. In the presence of the three factors above, a client is empowered to be autonomous in her care.

The role of health professionals in developing effective client self-care

It is important to make an assessment of the client's condition

a) What is the client's level of consciousness?

b) What is the client capable of doing in his state?

c) What are the client's needs?

d) How can the client achieve her needs?

It is important to decide what level of assistance the client needs. Conscious clients should be involved in the identification of their needs. Health personnel must choose appropriate methods of imparting the skills the client needs. It is important to discuss the methods with the client so that the client keeps up with what is happening. Adult education principles must be born in mind. Adults learn for immediate application of what they learn to their current situation especially to solve an immediate problem (Knowles et al.,1984; Brookfield,1986)

Knowledge needs

If the client needs knowledge, a decision must be made on whether to discuss with the client, the carer or relative or next of kin. Information must be given in manageable amounts that the client will be able to recall. It is important to always make available a leaflet that a client can refer to since clients do not take notes in the discussions with health personnel. What the client hears, she is likely to forget, the information may fade away with time and becomes distorted. Once the client forgets part of the information, she is likely to discard what remains of the information since it has gaps in the form of forgotten details. The client resorts to what she knows, what is known and believed around her, and what is accepted in her society.

Attitude change

If the client needs to change her attitude, health personnel should provide information in various forms to help the client to see facts from various angles. It must be remembered that behaviour emanates from strong attitudes and that attitudes are learnt, nurtured until they become values (Ajzen,1980). Attitudes develop over time and therefore attitudes take time to change (Ten Carte et al.,2000). Health personnel should not expect a change of attitude immediately after discussing a health issue with a client. Repeated discussions, allowing the client an opportunity to express their beliefs, fears and views and exchanging ideas and knowledge can help a client to appreciate new ideas and change attitudes. The client must be given leaflet with the same message contained in the subject of discussion to enable the client to internalise the message.

Acquisition of psychomotor skills

If the client requires psychomotor skills, it is important for health personnel to go through the activity with the client, repeat the procedure together with the client, asks the client to perform the skill while the health professional observes and advises. The client should repeat the procedure while the health professional observes. Repetition enhances learning (Darkenwald and Merriam,1982). Positive feedback acts as a re-enforcer for the client to learn more (Brookfield,1986). The health professional encourages the client to repeat the procedure repeatedly until the client masters the skill. The rule with psychomotor skills is 'We do it together, we repeat; you do it while I watch, Repeat, and continue to practice until you perfect your skills.' Many postnatal skills especially baby-care skills are learnt this way.

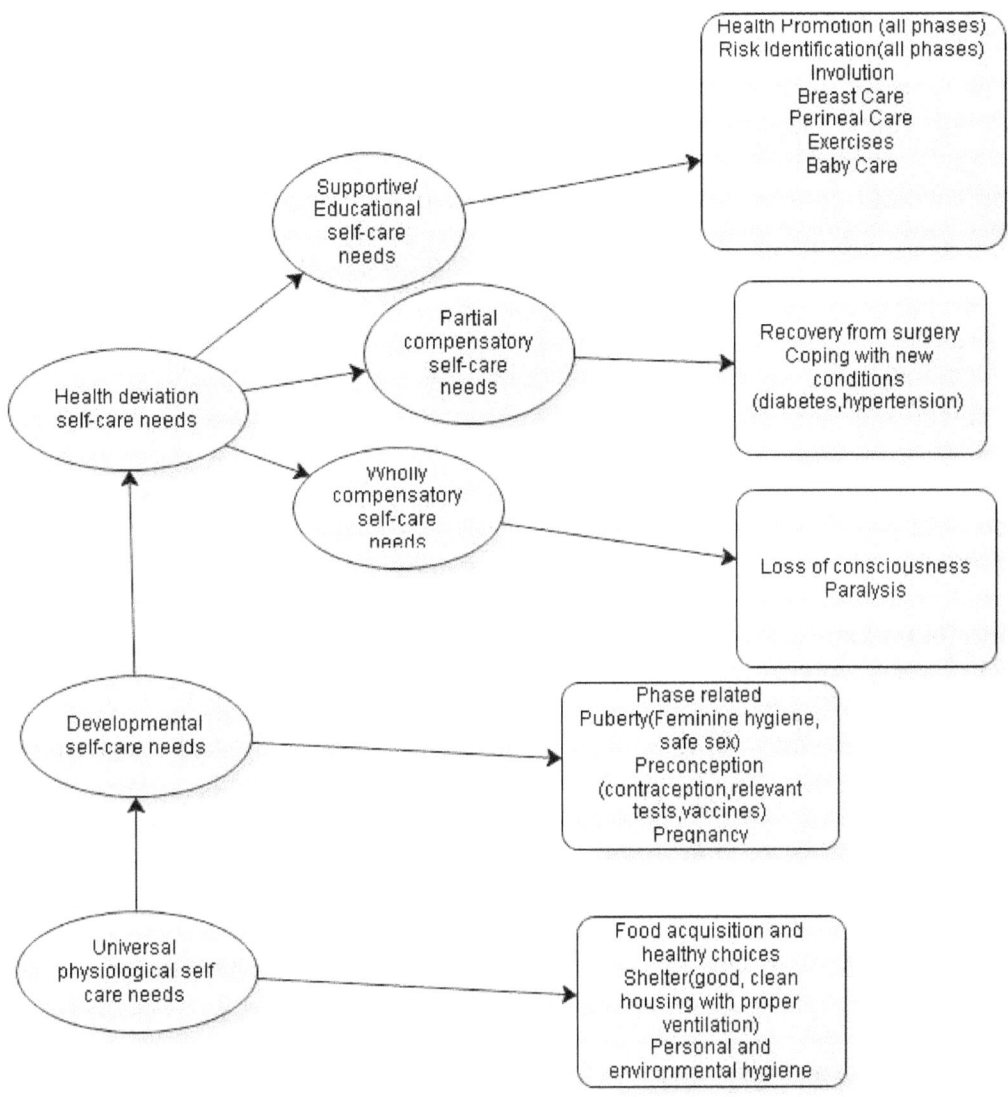

Fig. 6.2 **Self -care needs in reproductive health**

This figure explains the types of self-care and the levels or phases at which they are applicable in reproductive health.

Behavioural Theory

Health behaviour is influenced by the individual's knowledge of health, use of health information, and self-efficacy (Rimal, 2003). Clients without information may not necessarily be able to display or think about change of health behaviour without knowledge of the need to change. Without adequate information, clients may not have the confidence to try new health behaviours. Behavioural theorists have established that self efficacy has an impact on not only initiation of health behaviours but on behaviour maintenance (Rosenstock, 1966; Rosenstock et al., 1988; Maddux&Rogers, 1983; Ajzen, 1985; Bandura, 1995). Individuals with high self-efficacy are confident to engage in challenging health behaviours involving a change of their lifestyles while those with low self efficacy may have fear of failure (Maibach & Murphy, 1995).

Sexual and Reproductive Health Information given prior to and during each stage of the child bearing phase is likely to increase confidence and self efficacy in developing appropriate attitudes and behaviours among young women. According to the Social Learning Theory, behaviour change is determined by incentives, expectancies, benefits and capabilities to effect the change (Bandura, 1977). An expectant mother with hypertension might be more likely to comply with advice to rest *(behaviour)* if she understands and believes that rest will improve circulation to the placenta, and reduce the oedema of her ankles *(outcome/incentive)*, and if she believes that the "rest" will benefit her*(expectation)*and that she will be able to rest*(efficacy expectation).*

Health personnel have to explore factors that contribute to a client's perceived state of health, disease and risk in order to be able to facilitate the learning process, that eventually enables change of attitudes and behaviours among women (Naidoo&Wills, 2004;Ewles & Sinmet,1998).

The Behavioural Change Model (Prochaska& DiClemente, 1983, 1986, 1998)

This is a model that was initially used to observe behavioural change in smoking, alcohol and drug abuse, dietary changes and adherence to exercise and many other studies. The behavioural change model can also be applied to other behaviours including sexual and reproductive health behaviour change. Health personnel have to appreciate that the speed of behaviour change varies with individuals and the strength of their attitudes. The behavioural model utilizes strategies that encourage positive behaviour among individuals, families and communities in order for the people to adopt behaviours that promote healthy life styles. The individual has to take the initiative and decision to change behaviour while health personnel offer or create programmes and treatments that meet specific needs of each identified stage of behaviour.

The strength of the behavioural change model is that the client takes an active role in implementing the positive behaviour when they feel ready to do so. The driving force in one changing the behaviour is the availability of information and appreciation of the necessity to change behaviours. Clients must be provided with information as the first stage of the behavioural change but health personnel should not take it for granted that provision of information should bring about immediate change in women's behaviour because behavioural change is a process which proceeds through a series of stages. The client must understand how the proposed behaviours contribute towards good health as well as the consequences associated with ignoring the change of behaviour. Once one has adequate information, modification of behaviour may begin progressing through five stages as follows:

Pre-contemplation Stage: Clients are exposed to or sensitized to a problem through exposure to information. Many approaches to providing information are used so that a client has choice of a suitable source of information (word of mouth, discussion, leaflets, electronic media, observation of good behaviours).The presence of information alone should not be expected to bring about or cause intention to change.

Contemplation Stage The client is aware that a problem exists. The client may be planning change at some time to come. There is no commitment to change as yet and the individual has not yet thought how they may bring about this change (Bennet & Murphy, 1997). Midwives must appreciate that understanding and appreciating information does not occur at the same rate in clients. For some clients, it takes a while to change attitudes especially if the client is surrounded by family and community with strong cultural beliefs and values.

Preparation Stage There is a strong attitude and an intention to change behaviour and the client plans to effect the change of behaviour. The client begins to make preparation for the change. The client contemplates on change of behaviour based on awareness of the consequences of her behaviour and the outcome expectancies (Fishbein & Ajzen, 1975; 1980). Most action is under voluntary control and largely guided by intention. Intention is driven by strong attitudes and the influence of significant others, peer pressure, media influence, socio-economic and political context (Bennet & Murphy, 1997). Behavioural change includes the process of empowerment, which reduces reliance on and control by other people.

Action Stage: The client modifies her way of life and environment to allow for change of behaviour. It however requires at least two months of maintaining behavioural change for it to be considered true behavioural change. Some people tend to relapse and give up as soon as they meet with hurdles in their efforts or as soon as they feel the difficulty of this behaviour modification undoing the positive progress they may have achieved. Primiparous women may meet with more hurdles as they may be believed by their society to be inexperienced and without decision making powers. They will therefore require continuous support from health personnel once they decide to take action to change their behaviours.

Maintenance: The individual resolves to prevent relapse and works towards achievement of their goal. Schwarzer, (1992) attributes the effort to maintain behaviours on a type of environment the person is exposed to and the social support one has which is important complementary factors to behaviour change.

Behavioural change is therefore a long process the results of which should not be expected immediately after a single lecture but after a period of sustained information giving and continued support to the clients.

Health promotion action in sexual and reproductive health includes a new and demanding role for midwives; that of continuous lobbying and advocacy for the needs of women Midwives must continuously be conscious and alert and make a critical analysis of women's health policies put in place in order to assess and measure their impact on the women's health (Bunton & McDonald, 2002; Harrison, 2002). Lobbying and advocacy on behalf of marginalised clients are important skills that midwives and other health personnel should develop and these require good communication skills

The social cognitive theory (Bandura, 1977; 1986) suggests that individuals respond to external stimuli by actively participating through observations. Retention and producing behaviours is based on one's self-efficacy and environmental influences and influences of social circles such as the young modelling what the elder members of society do. The social change approach aims at modifying people's environment and socio-economic status in order to improve health, so that the healthy choices become the obvious reasonable choices (Ewles and Simnet, 1998; Naidoo& Orme, 2000; Naidoo & Wills, 2004). There is need for health personnel to appreciate the groups that make up a particular society they serve, their culture, beliefs and values, their knowledge, health concerns and the meaning of health to the people.

Health promotion is the linchpin to empowering women with information that enables them to understand good health, understand the normal woman's health and enables them to identify abnormal features to their health or risks to their health.

References

1. Ajzen, I. and Madden, T.J. (1986). Prediction of goal directed behaviour: attitudes intentions and perceived behavioural control. *Journal of Experimental Social Psychology*. 22, pp. 435-474.

2. Ajzen, I. and Fishbein, M. (1980). *Understanding attitudes and predicting social behaviour*. New Jersey: Prentice Hall.

3. Bandura, A. (1995). *Self-efficacy in changing societies*. New York: Cambridge University Press.

4. Bandura, A. (1986). *Social foundations of thought and action*. Englewood Cliffs, NJ: Prentice Hall.

5. Bandura, A. (1977). *Social learning theory*. Englewood Cliffs, NJ: Prentice Hall Brookfield, S.D. (1986). *Understanding and Facilitating Adult Learning*. Milton Keynes: Open University Press.

6. Burnett, P. and Murphy, S. (1997). *Psychology and Health Promotion*. Buckingham: Open University Press.

7. Bunton, R. and Macdonald, G. (2002). *Health Promotion. Disciplines, diversity and developments*. London: Routledge.

8. Comeley, A.L. (1994). A comparative analysis of Orem's self-care model and Peplau's Interpersonal theory. *Journal of Advanced Nursing*. 20, pp. 755-760.

9. Darkenwald, G.G. and Merriam,S.B.Adult Education: Foundations of Practice. New York. Harper & Row,1982

10. Ewles, L. and Simnett, I. (1999). *Promoting health: a practice guide*. 4th ed. Edinburgh: Bailliere Tindall.

11. Harrison, D. (2002). Health promotion and the politics of integration. In: Bunton, R., Macdonald, G. and Bunton, P. *Health Promotion: Disciplines, diversity and developments*. 2nd ed. London: Routledge.

12. Fishbein, M. (1993). Introduction. In: Terry, D.J., Gallois, C. and McCamish, M. *The theory of reasoned action: Its application to AIDS preventive behaviour*. Oxford: Pergamon Press.

13. Fishbein, M. and Ajzen, I. (1995). *Belief, Attitude, Intention and Behaviour*. New York: John Wiley.

14. Knowles,M.S.,and Associates.Andragogy in Action. Applying Modern Principles of Adult LearningSan Francisco:Jossey –Bass, 1984.

15. Maddux, J.E. and Rogers, R.W. (1983). Protection Motivation and self-efficacy: a revised theory of fear appeals and attitude change. *Journal of Experimental Social Psychology*. 19, pp. 469-479.

16. Maslow, A. (1971). *Motivation and Personality*. New York: Harper & Row.

17. Naidoo, J. and Wills, J. (2004). *Health Promotion: Foundations for Practice*. 2nd Ed. Edinburgh: Bailliere Tindall.

18. Naidoo, J. and Orme, J. (2000). Health promotion in the medical curriculum: enhancing its potential. *Medical Teacher*. 22(3), pp. 282-287.

19. Orem, D.E.(1985)Nursing: Concepts of Practice 3rd ed. Mcgraw Hill, New York.

20. Prochaska, J.O. and DiClemente, C.C. (1986). Towards a comprehensive model of change. In: Miller, W.R. and Heather, N. *Treating addictive behaviours*. 2nd ed. New York: Plenum.

21. Prochaska, J.O., DiClemente, C.C. and Norcross, J.C. (1992). In search of how people change: applications to addictive behaviours. *American Psychologist*. 47, pp. 1102-1114.

22. Rimal, R.N. (2003). Intergenerational Transmission of Health: The role of intrapersonal, interpersonal and Communicative Factors. *Health Education and Behaviour*. 30(1), pp. 10-28.

23. Rosenstock, I.M. (1966). Why people use health services. *The Milibank Memorial Fund Quarterly*. 44(3), pp. 94-124.

24. Rosenstock, I.R. (1990). The Health Belief Model: Explaining Health Behaviour through expectancies. In: Glantnz, K. *Health behaviour and health education: theory, research, and practice*. San Francisco: Jossey-Bass, pp. 39-62.

25. Schwarzer, R. (1992). Self-efficacy in the adoption and maintenance of health behaviours: theoretical approaches and a new model. In: Schwarzer, R. *Self-efficacy: Thought control of action*. Washington DC: Hemisphere.

26. ten Cate, Th.J. and de Haes, J.C.J.M. (2000). Summative assessment of medical students in the affective domain. *Medical Teacher*. 22(1), pp. 40-43.

CHAPTER 7

MENTAL STATE OF THE MOTHER POST DELIVERY

The child bearing experience and the subsequent new responsibilities are huge changes that emerge within a very short space of each other. Many young women need support to enable them to gradually ease into their new roles. There are physical, mental, social and environmental challenges a new mother may encounter and these require that she be able to adapt to them before they become stressors (Detherage et al.,2005) Some young women may adjust well and grasp their responsibilities with enthusiasm but there are some who can be shaken and overwhelmed by the whole experience that comes as a shock surpassing their expectations. Some young women may be overwhelmed and may view motherhood as a mammoth task. Some young mothers may find the experience shocking and surpassing their expectations. Some women may have a feeling of inadequacy, helplessness that may invoke some distress.

Triggers of Distress

a)Unmet Expectations

Post delivery, a woman can be depressed by lack of support from the spouse due to unmet expectations resulting in withdrawal of support. In some cultures baby boys are still valued more than baby girls. A woman delivering a baby girl where a baby boy would have been preferred may meet with unexpected lack of support from a spouse. Controversy on the age of pregnancy where paternity of the baby is doubted has been reported to cause distress to a new mother. It is important that health personnel find time to discuss with a young woman displaying signs of stress to identify the possible and probable root of the problem. Possible interventions can then be put into place to resolve the cause of the stress in the best possible way.

b) Single parenthood and lack of Family Support

Extreme stressful situations in pregnancy have been associated with distress triggering puerperal psychosis in some cases. Murira,(2010) reports on poor family support in primiparous women who were jilted by their lovers in pregnancy and had babies out of wedlock. The young women filled with shame,fear and distress developed severe puerperal psychosis in the first week post delivery.

Single parenthood is a difficult situation which usually has social and economic implications that will need to be discussed and a possible solution devised. Lack of support spousal and family support may be responsible for baby dumping, infanticide and puerperal psychosis. The young woman must be assisted to piece her life together gradually. Provision of intensive post partum support by midwives has been identified as a useful intervention (Dennis &Creedy, 2004). A prescription of anti-depressants on its own is not adequate in puerperal psychosis. Getting over puerperal psychosis is a process that requires patience on the part of health personnel and dialogue with the affected woman and her immediate carers. This cannot be achieved in one or two visits. Where possible a psychologist and social worker should be summoned to assist the client to accept her situation and help her plan her future. Such a client should be followed up over a prolonged period until the health personnel are satisfied that she has recovered from her trauma and is focussed on building her life afresh.

c)Operative delivery

Operative delivery is viewed differently from one society to the other. While some societies may prefer an operative delivery to the pain of labour, an operative delivery may be shunned in other societies. Some women may feel inadequate and may consider themselves failures or a disgrace to be delivered by Caesarean Section. Some cultures associate operative delivery with an evil spell and may live under the fear of having been bewitched. Health personnel should be at hand to provide counselling to the spouse and members of the family. In some cultures, failure to deliver the first baby normally is associated with failure to disclose other previous sexual partners. It is important that health personnel are familiar with local beliefs so that they can provide effective relevant antenatal education that is culture centred, as well as counselling and scientific explanations to events of pregnancy and labour to counter locally held beliefs.

d)Insufficient Rest

A new baby brings joy to new parents and yet the arrival of the baby may mean reduced sleep hours, reduced leisure time during the day for the new mother and a general increase in the chores that must be attended to by the new mother. Lack of rest may cause extreme exhaustion, pyrexia, poor healing of wounds, poor lactation and poor sleep patterns. Insufficient rest can be taxing on the new mother. Couples need to be familiar with baby care skills and counselled on sharing baby care chores before the baby arrives and after the baby has arrived to encourage partners to develop confidence to participate fully in the care of the baby. Couples can be advised to seek help from a friend or relative if possible, or engage hired help to assist with chores.

e)Perineal Injury

Pain and poor healing of the perineal area is a major source of discomfort and distress post delivery. Excessive perineal oedema may occur where stitches are too tight and cut deep into the flesh making walking and sitting extremely difficult and painful. Sometimes it may be necessary to release one or two interrupted stitches to give the woman some relief. Episiotomies and perineal tears in some societies are associated with failure to make adequate preparations for labour and delivery. A young woman with perineal trauma may be associated with failure to comply with tradition and may be pushed into depression and psychosis.

It may be necessary for the health visitor to assist the woman with vulval toilet using recommended antiseptics to clear slough away in the case of broken down episiotomy, until the wound is clean and ready for secondary suturing or shows signs of healing. Some women are depressed by the stretch of the birth canal during delivery and fear that their birth canals will never be the same.

A repaired vulva has some discomfort that a woman has to contend with and that can interfere with smooth return to normal activity for some time. It is important that the health visitor and the client have an open discussion about such discomfort and the woman is made aware of the source of the discomfort and reassured that it will disappear with time.

Fistulae

A fistula is an opening between two organs such as between the uterus and the bladder, between the uterus and the large bowel , and between the large bowel, uterus and bladder. A fistula occurs as a result of obstructed labour and delay in seeking health care services in contracted pelvis, abnormal fetal lie, large baby, extensive female circumcision and genital mutilation. This birth trauma is preventable if awareness of importance of antenatal care is created in communities and women have access to prompt medical attention(Gessessew & Melese,2002; Ogunnowo et al 2003; Odusoga et al,2003). Vesico-vaginal fistula and recto-vaginal fistula may be a thing of the past in some parts of the world, but these may still be fairly common in some developing countries. The causes may also vary from one community to the other. Whatever the causes, fistulae erode the dignity and confidence of a woman. A fistula causes untold distress and desperation as the woman battles against, the loss of function of her most feminine parts of her body, the uncontrolled linkage of wastes and the related odour and stigma, and worse still, the inevitable deterioration of relationships with her partner. The distress is usually compounded by the fact that fistulae in most cases are associated with fetal loss. The woman so affected has to be handled with a lot of sympathy and empathy. She needs information on how to cope with her situation, to include feminine hygiene. She needs to be informed at each stage of management the objectives and benefits of each step taken. She needs to be informed of how she can participate in self-care to speed up recovery. She also needs information on diet, family planning and prevention of recurrence of condition through use of available health services like antenatal clinics and waiting shelters with subsequent pregnancies. The partner needs to be counselled and involved in the management of his spouse and the relevant health education.

Bereavement

Common causes of bereavement are

Loss of a pregnancy through abortion, miscarriage, intrauterine death, stillbirth,

Loss of a child as in neonatal death

A baby with a congenital abnormality

Loss of fertility as in salpingectomy and hysterectomy

Signs of Stress

Close observation of the behaviour of the mother and discussion with her helps to assess her mental state and reveal some underlying emotions likely to cause depression. A postnatal mother who displays or is reported to have some of or all of the signs below needs to be watched closely. New mothers have some form of anxiety about the baby that may cause them to want to check on the baby repeatedly but this has to be closely watched. a) Sleep disturbances, such as short episodes of sleep and long periods of sleeplessness This may be an early warning sign of an ensuing depression.

a) Fatigue, and difficulty in concentration, failing to keep a straight line of conversation, or constantly talking to self.

b) Refusal to feed the baby, dislike for the baby, displayed in many ways like staring at the baby while the baby cries, shouting at or screaming at the baby to keep quiet, holding the baby tightly and shaking the baby, threatening to get rid of the baby and many odd behaviours that do not display love, is certainly depressed.

c) Neglect of personal hygiene such as failure to change sanitary towels, failure to change soiled clothes or take a bath is a sign of depression.

d) Irritability, weepy new mother who feels unwanted and worthless

e) A mother who isolates herself or becomes withdrawn could be depressed and may develop puerperal psychosis(Davidhizar&Giger,1994)

f) A mother who identifies one person that she hates most often feeling agitated in that person's presence is in a state of depression.

g) Restlessness and failure to settle down for any basic chores expected of a mother.

h) A mother who hears voices or talks to herself is on the verge of psychosis.

i) Attempting to harm the baby or desert the baby. Some depressed women have been known to want to strangle babies or throw them out through windows.

j) Inappropriate handling of the baby as if the baby were a doll or any other object A depressed woman may forget that she has a baby and some may fail to realise that they are holding a baby preferring to clutch the baby like a handbag.

k) Aggression and lack of cooperation is common and may be a reaction to previous events in the family or an underlying worrying problem. She may become violent with other clients, or may be accusatory.

l) Loss of appetite is almost always present in a woman with psychosis, with the woman completely ignoring the food or nibbling it or just playing with it, mixing it but not eating it.

A woman with puerperal psychosis may have some of the above signs in varying degrees.

What is Postnatal Depression?

Postnatal depression may include several symptoms observed in a newly delivered mother for at least two to three weeks for a diagnosis to be made(Musters et al.,2009). Some of the symptoms are a depressed mood

Puerperal psychosis is a mental health problem that occurs in the first few days after delivery of a baby. Puerperal psychosis is associated with some potential risk factors such as recent stressful events like the process of childbirth, poor social support, lack of supportive partner and a history of other psychiatric conditions as well as heredity (Musters et al., 2009). This condition contributes to severe distress among primiparous women post delivery. The conditions are made worse by strong, negative unsympathetic attitudes and beliefs about mental illness prevalent within close family and society as a whole.

Puerperal psychosis is not fully understood in many African societies. Family members may regard the mental illness as a curse that requires spiritual cultural cleansing rituals and these cultural rituals seem to be the accepted management of puerperal psychosis in the Shona society (Murira,2010). Various rituals are enacted in some cultures in an attempt to correct the situation. The lack of knowledge about the cause of puerperal psychosis and the management of the condition negatively affects care and support of the young women affected. Disturbing observations where women are isolated from the rest of the family and society in locked up rooms to prevent them from disturbing the rest of the family and bringing shame to the family have been noted.

A high rate of early onset of puerperal psychosis in young primiparous women was reported in Tanzania even where there was post partum support from family members, suggesting that there is more to prevention of puerperal psychosis than family support alone (Ndosi & Mtawali 2002).

Managing a woman with postnatal depression

The depressed and withdrawn mother may not be easy to deal with, as the cause for her withdrawal may not be readily known. Patience in dealing with such a mother is necessary.

a) It is important to maintain respect for the client and accept her position.

b) Health personnel should invite and initiate discussion and ask the mother to communicate her problems. The client should be allowed to vent her feelings and must be patiently given time to settle. She can then be invited to discuss the source of her anger.

c) Avoid taking sides or justifying certain actions. The ability of the health visitor to handle emotional encounters is enhancing and enabling in the provision of care. Explanation is best done when the anger is diffused.

It may take a while before the woman decides to talk. The woman will talk if she trusts the health professional and is not hurried.

One research compared the incidence of puerperal psychosis in primiparous women who had attended antenatal exercises and those who had not. The results were inconclusive about the role of antenatal exercise in reducing postnatal depression (Daley et al., 2009).

Although some researchers suggest that use of anti-depressants may reduce puerperal psychosis, there are sentiments that prescriptions on their own may not adequately manage puerperal psychosis as there are socio-cultural issues to consider in puerperal psychosis. There is therefore a suggestion that both family support and intensive post -partum support by health professionals like the community psychiatric nurses, and psychologists are useful interventions in prevention and management of puerperal psychosis (Dennis & Creedy, 2004).

Breaking Bad News

A mother who has lost a pregnancy, a baby before delivery, during delivery or after delivery should have this news appropriately delivered to her. In circumstances where the bad news is impending such as in premature labour, a very ill neonate, the mother and her spouse must be informed of the condition and informed at each stage of care about the changes in condition, All efforts that are being made to rectify the situation must be known to all concerned. This is useful in the event of failure to save the pregnancy or the infant or the mother that the next of kin should have been prepared for it. Breaking bad news is a process and not a one off event (Harden,1996). Part of this process is preparing a woman and her spouse of the inevitable by keeping them informed of the events as they unfold. The parents of an ill baby should be informed of what measures are being taken and what the prognosis is so that should the ill baby suddenly stop breathing, parents should not be taken by surprise as the condition will have been explained before hand. A clear explanation of the possible causes of death in the case of a baby collapsing should help the bereaved parents go through their loss with full information that the best was tried to save life. It must be remembered that pregnancy loss or neonatal death affects the mother physically, psychologically and emotionally and may have an impact on subsequent pregnancies. A woman who has had a stillbirth preterm labour, low birth weight baby, placental abruption with the rate of another stillbirth increased up to ten times (Reddy,2007). A multidisciplinary counselling about the cause of the loss and support for the couple must be arranged. The presence of a support person, although ideal, may not be possible all the time, but where a relative, spouse is available, they should be involved. Finding the cause of the loss and involving clients helps in the management of future pregnancies and helps parents to go through the grieving process and quickly come to a closure (Tiegen,2008).

How to break bad news

A quiet environment without the disturbances of the telephone and other activities would be an ideal place in which to break the bad news.

Health personnel must share emotions with the client and express their condolences to the bereaved. This breaks down barriers and shows that health personnel are human. Sharing emotions breaks down social barriers (Graham,1991). Failure to show compassion may be seen by the bereaved as arrogance and being impersonal. Bad news must be given slowly ; it should never be rushed since the client needs time to take in the news and react. It is necessary to repeat this process when the spouse or relatives are present. If the telling process is not repeated, a client may refuse to accept the explanation given. The client looks for someone to blame for the loss of her loved one. It is best that follow up meetings/visits be made to create opportunities for the parents to ask questions and perhaps request the initial discussion in full. This helps parents in the process of grieving to slowly assimilate the information and accept their plight. Acceptance gives them the drive to carry on and look to the future.

Expression of feelings may range from a complete silence to quiet sobs or a hysteric outburst. Some clients may ask to be left alone for a while. Some may ask several questions, while others are so shocked that they fail to say anything. When they are ready to ask questions, it is important that their questions are responded to as honestly as possible.
It is unethical to give false hopes e.g." All will be well" when the prognosis is poor.
Or "We just hope for the best", when it is obvious that the condition is not compatible with life. Clear explanation of the condition if it interferes with normal life should be provided.

Use of illustrations where possible to explain the body system and provide a clear picture in simple everyday language is advised. If there are alternatives these should be made known to the client or next of kin.

Who Should Break Bad News

All health personnel should be able to break bad news(Couper,1994) Ideally, the person breaking the news should be familiar to the client, it could be the doctor, or the midwife, who knows about the client and the events leading to the death, or to the loss of organ or familiar with the abnormality. Ideally all health professionals should have the skills to break bad news. A radiographer who diagnoses intrauterine death on ultrasound scan should be able to break the news to the client, and sends the client to the doctor for further management. In the event of a loss of life, it is professional and moral that the team of health professionals who has been looking after the client deal with the bereaved, conveying condolences and answering questions from the bereaved.

Maternal Feelings After a Loss

After a loss, the couple, especially the woman often feels shocked, devastated and frustrated about the loss. They may have anger at loosing the pregnancy and may be full of self-accusation and guilt that probably they are to blame for the loss. Some women maybe full of despair and apprehension that they may never achieve another successful pregnancy again. Many may blame others especially health personnel especially in such cases as fresh stillbirth and neonatal death. There is always the assumption that the pregnancy or neonate could have been saved had health personnel done what they failed to do. All mothers who lost wanted pregnancies and babies are sorrowful and may weep incessantly. Health personnel looking after such clients should be sensitive to the client's situation and manage each client as an individual whose reaction to the loss may be different from any other woman. Mothers often feel shocked and distraught after their loss (Weiss,1987).

Critical Incident

Mrs. Zero delivered a live female infant who subsequently died within 24hours after delivery. On the home visit, Mrs. Zero sobbed uncontrollably and accused the doctor, the midwife and her colleagues who had attended to her at the hospital of poor communication, gross negligence and responsible for the death of her baby.

Care After Loss

Health personnel should show compassion and empathy. The presence of someone all the time is important in case the woman wants to talk makes a lot of difference. Parents can be assisted not forced to see the baby even in the case of gross abnormality. The baby should be properly wrapped and handed to them. They may take their time to view the baby but will eventually do so. If the parents so wish, a hospital chaplain can be contacted to baptize the baby or just to pray with them. Photographs can be taken if the parents so wish. Death registration and disposal of the baby should be discussed and consent obtained from both parents for this. The choice of the parents prevails all the time. Counseling sessions should start immediately. The spouse should be included.In the first hour or two, the mother may not want to talk but the presence of someone, a member of the health team, just in case the mother may want to talk, makes a difference.

A caring touch on the hand, an arm around the shoulders means as much as words, as long as one understands the culture and selects an acceptable mode of touch (Ojanlatva,1994).In the presence of a caring person, a grieving mother sooner or later may want to express herself verbally through some conversation. Help through a conversation should never be under estimated. After a loss, a mother should preferably be afforded continuity of care preferably by someone they met earlier on so that the mother is not continuously being reminded of her loss by new faces asking about the baby or the pregnancy. Where this is not possible, health professionals must make an effort to read details of their clients from the notes on the ward before meeting them and not make assumptions that all women in the ward have had successful pregnancy outcomes.

Counselling sessions should be commenced as early as possible. The spouse should be included in the discussion. The spouse's loss must be acknowledged and should be given his space for grieving. Parents can be helped not forced to see the baby even in the case of gross deformity. The baby should be properly wrapped and handed to them. Once the baby is handed to them, they may take their time to view the baby but will eventually do so. Removing the baby too quickly from the ward makes it difficult for the young and nervous couples who may be unsure initially if they want to see their baby, but may change their minds later.

Some institutions have come up with "A Chapel of Rest", a room where the dead babies can be kept for a while in case the parents want to have a look again. Parents can be encouraged to give the baby a name. Many couples will have decided on a name earlier on during pregnancy.

A hospital chaplain can be contacted to baptize the baby if the parents so wish. Parents can take photographs of their child if they wish. Some institutions do this routinely and keep one photograph for the records while the other photograph is given to parents. However parents can be allowed to take a photograph of their baby. Death registration and disposal of the baby should be discussed and consent obtained from both parents.

Room Choice

Mothers must be asked where they prefer to stay after a loss. Preferably she must be nursed in an environment that does not constantly remind her of her loss. Women have been reported to feel comfortable nursed in gynaecology wards or side rooms where every woman is experiencing a loss of one type or another. It may be easier for them to unwind and talk about their loss freely as well as make friends with other women also in the same position.

Mothers who have lost a pregnancy or a baby should be asked where they prefer to stay postnatally. Some women may find the postnatal ward uncomfortable as it constantly reminds them of their loss. The closeness to success will constantly remind them of their failure. The cry of babies and meeting mothers with successful pregnancy outcomes, the happiness that prevails in corridors especially during visiting time may be depressing. It can be difficult to interact with others who are not similarly affected.

The stay in the postnatal ward or side ward in a maternity ward may stir deep emotions that are difficult to deal with as described by one woman with gestational diabetes after delivering a fresh stillborn baby.

Critical incident

" All seemed well until that fateful morning. I could not feel any fetal movements. I was rushed to theatre for a Caesarean section but the baby was already dead at caesarean Section. I was initially nursed in a ward. There were four of us who had had operations, except that the other three women had their babies there with them. I kept on hoping that the midwife or the doctor would come and tell me that my baby was alive. My baby had looked so healthy and beautiful it was hard to believe he was dead. I could not sleep except when I was under heavy sedation. The woman next to me kept on talking loudly to her baby as if to tease me. The visiting times were the most difficult. You could tell the other women had whispered something to their visitors by the way everyone looked at me. I preferred to cover my head and not see the happy faces across. Every time a baby cried, I also cried with grief. I felt so frustrated I wished I could leave the hospital. But I had to stay on since I had a fresh wound. I was still on treatment for diabetes and my blood sugar was still quite high. I picked up courage and asked the midwives if they could change my bed. I was moved into a side room. For a day I was alone. It was a relief but very lonely. It was as if I had been forgotten there. I couldn't stop crying. When my partner came visiting, we both cried throughout the visiting time. After my partner left, I was devastated. It seemed I could not completely escape from the rejoicing voices in the corridors and the baby talk in the communal bathrooms. Somehow at the change of shifts, there was always one member of hospital staff among those coming on duty that did not know about my plight and asked me about the baby. It was a painful reminder to have to explain all the time that I had lost my baby."

The Antenatal Side-room An antenatal side-room can be very lonely. Side-rooms as a whole no matter which set up there are in can be very lonely and eerie after a loss. Health care staff tends to be hesitant to frequent the side-room. It could be to give the mother a quiet time, but the mother may feel forgotten.

The Gynaecology ward

Some bereaved mothers may find the gynaecology ward a safe hideaway and very appropriate because everyone in the ward has no success story to talk about. There are no embarrassing questions asked about the baby. Women can talk about their feelings freely without offending someone or without the occasional cry of the baby and baby language

Arrangements must be made for continuous moral support of the bereaved mother through home visits. It is important that the bereaved mother is sent home to a supportive environment. A health visitor, and a psychologist monitor the bereaved mother closely until all signs of mental depression have cleared.

After the loss of a baby, the mother recalls every detail. The thoughts of such an event will linger on for many years to come. She went through all the feelings of expectation and anticipation. She went through a lot of imagination of herself after the arrival of the baby. She had a name ready for the baby. She had bought clothes for the unborn baby in anticipation. The baby's place in the home is ready. The mother went through the process of labour and hoped to have a live baby. Suddenly the baby died. The feeling is like a bad dream, a theft, the most painful experience a woman can ever encounter.

This deep grief will bring the baby's cry unconsciously in the mother's ears. A live baby is what she expected and during this critical period, her thoughts are turned into her expectations. She also dreams about the baby and may wake up to look for the baby only to realize it was a dream. This is an experience most women who have lost babies relate.

"Every time I go to sleep I wake up often because I hear my baby crying." (Murira, 2010)

In the state of anguish after a loss of a baby or a pregnancy, clients expect health personnel to show compassion during the process of grieving. Clients expect to be told the truth and given an opportunity to share emotions. Failure to show emotions is seen by clients as insensitive and inhuman. A bereaved mother must receive support and attention. All staff attending to her must be empathetic towards her. At the same time, she must be urged to look ahead and carry on with life. Her concerns must be listened to and she must be involved in working out a solution. She needs people with patience and willingness to listen as she pours out her grief. Talking to an attentive audience is a form of self- therapy and it brings closure to the loss quickly. After a loss of a baby, women need a lot of support from both the health care team and the relatives until they pass through this period of denial and reach a period of rationalising in the grieving process.

Although anti-depressants may be prescribed, they should be seen as complimentary to the social support. Without good social support a woman may break down and develop a serious psychiatric problem.

Other circumstances

There can be other circumstances in the home that can cause untold discomfort in a newly delivered mother and if not identified and attended to, can lead to puerperal psychosis.

Mrs. Lemon left hospital having delivered a baby boy two days before. She lived with her husband in a one bed roomed apartment in the city. When the midwife arrived to visit, Mrs. Lemon was crying, baby in hands. The midwife thought that since this was Mrs. Lemon's first baby, Mrs. Lemon may have had problems with fixing the baby to the breast, she could have been in pain, she could have engorged breasts, a painful episiotomy or simply could not cope with her new responsibility. After discussing with her, it was discovered that while she had many other minor problems, her major worry was her husband. Mr. Lemon could not stand the cry of the baby. He could not look at the baby feeding. He threw up a tantrum in the presence of the midwife and threatened to throw the baby out through the window. After a long discussion with the midwife, Mr. Lemon revealed that he had been treated for a psychiatric disorder a few years back, but had stopped the medication when he got better. He had not informed his wife about his previous medical problem.

In this situation, neither the obstetrician nor the midwife would have guessed that such a situation would arise. A weepy new mother almost always has a major problem that can be missed if the health visitor does not take time to listen to the mother and study the environment in which the mother and her baby are in.

Understanding Clients Culture It is imperative that health personnel are familiar with their clients' culture and religion to enable them to offer culturally acceptable care following a loss. Health personnel should not question clients' beliefs (Heazell & McLaughlin, 2010). It is also important to understand a woman's culture to enable one to appreciate the connotations of a pregnancy loss in a particular culture in order to offer relevant health information and health education. In the African culture, women fall pregnant for various reasons. Some women fall pregnant to secure a marriage, to consolidate a marriage, to get an heir in the family, to get company and to get respect as adults in the society. For many women, once they discover that they are pregnant, whether the pregnancy is planned or not, they are happy to carry the pregnancy to term. Loss of a pregnancy for many women is devastating. In the event of loosing a pregnancy, women have a right to be treated as individuals and not routinely. The health professionals should apply good clinician-client relationship with the client and communicate all the relevant information about investigations and procedures after a loss to dispel rumours and suspicions associated with such procedures like post mortem.

Essential information

Following a loss, mothers go through a normal puerperium as their counterparts with successful pregnancy outcomes.Information on lactation and care of the breasts to prevent breast complications post delivery should be made available.

Women may be anxious to fall pregnant immediately to forget the loss. Information on the need for the body to recuperate and other pre-conceptual information before another pregnancy is essential. It is important to advise the clients on the importance of enabling the body to recover before falling pregnant again following an abortion, a miscarriage or a neonatal loss. This is more so especially in those cultures, which believe in a mother replacing the lost pregnancy immediately to avert loneliness and depression. Effective family planning methods must be discussed with the couple. Information on the importance of early booking for antenatal services when another pregnancy does occur is imparted.

Information on the importance of early booking for antenatal services when another pregnancy has occurred is imparted.

Counselling is necessary where the loss was due to gross abnormality incompatible with life in full term pregnancy. In genetic abnormalities, genetic counselling should be commenced immediately. The couple are given time to moan over their loss and arrangements made for follow up visits and further counselling. Where a pregnancy has been lost through an abortion and miscarriage, details of the events prior to the abortion or miscarriage must be obtained to form a basis for client education and counselling. Information on support groups in the case of congenital abnormalities should be made available to the couple.

Information on support groups where available should be made available to the couple. A support group could be formed by such people as the midwife, the health visitor, a psychologist, an obstetrician, a paediatrician, a hospital chaplain and a GP, to discuss any problems and requests that bereaved mothers may have. This can help to allay fears and misconceptions that may be present within the bereaved mothers. The meetings help the mothers to network with others in the same predicament and this is a healing process in itself.The possible stress and strain on the marriage and siblings after a loss should be discussed. Marriages have been known to dissipate due to repeated pregnancy loss.

Discharge home should be on an individual basis. Some mothers may be very lonely at home and may wish to stay for a day longer or until they have made arrangements for company at home.

The mother can be forewarned on the reaction of neighbours and other pregnant women neighbours who may not feel comfortable in her presence and may tend to avoid her. Some of the reactions may be due to uncertainty of what to say in her presence while some pregnant mothers may react that way out of superstition and desire to "protect" their pregnancies from evil spells.

A discharge Planner should be made to the health visitor who should constantly monitor the mother's recovery process and offer professional support. Some mothers may wish to stay a day longer or until they have made arrangements about a social support at home. A psychologist should continue to visit the mother until the health care team is satisfied with the physical and mental state of the mother. Postnatal support should include advice on other activities in life like a new hobby, skill acquisition or joining a club to help the process of emotional healing.

Q.E.1)To what extent are the above ideas applicable in your situation?2)Plan a programme of care for your bereaved clients using guidelines from the above ideas taking into consideration the culture of your clientele, and resources available.3)How are bereaved mothers in your organization managed. Compare the ideas in this module and the practice in your institution.4)Find out what bereaved mothers in your community think about your management of the bereaved.

Loss of an Organ

Clients may end up with unexpected removal of organs in emergency operations such as salpingectomy following an ectopic abortion, or hysterectomy following a ruptured uterus. It is imperative that couples are given full information of what the operation entailed and that they are counselled. It is unethical for health personnel to fail to give the full information of such operations and the consequences of the operations, as this is part of truth telling and professional ethics that health personnel must observe in offering health care services(Hope e al.,2004). Information on physiological changes as a result of the emergency removal of organs such as cessation of menses and fertility after the removal of the uterus, for instance, must be explained. Couples must be given full information of the differences between total hysterectomy and partial and reassurances that organ loss will not affect sexual relationships. The women should undergo thorough counselling to include subsequent feeling of anxiety, inadequacy, unworthiness and embarrassment that women may feel after organ loss. It is important that follow up meetings in which women can express their anxieties and problems are planned as part of post natal care and counselling.

Maternal Death

Where maternal death occurs, the spouse must be given an opportunity to understand clearly events leading to the death of the partner. Follow up meetings must be arranged where the process of explanation must be repeated to ease the grieving process. Where a mother leaves behind a live baby and siblings, efforts must be made to assist with information that enables the best possible care of the baby. The health visitor must continue to visit and monitor the care of the baby. The social worker must be actively involved too.

Reference

1.Couper,I. Medical students' attitudes towards death and related issues.S.A.Family Practice.1994 (!5) 505-511

2.Daley, A., Jolly, K. and Macarthur C. (2009). The effectiveness of exercise in the Management of postnatal depression: systematic review and meta-analysis. *Family Practitioner*. 26(2), pp. 154-162.

3. Davidhizar, R. & Giger, J.N. When your patient is silent. Journal of Advanced Nursing, 1994,(20) 703-706

Dennis, C.L., and Creedy, D. (2004). Psychosocial and psychological interventions for Preventing postnatal depression. *Cochrane Database of Systematic Reviews*. (4), CD001134.

4.Detherage,K.S;Johnson,S.S;Mandle,L.C. Stress Management and Crisis intervention in Edelman and Mandle, Health Promotion along the life-line (2005)pp299-310

5.Gessessew, A. and Melese, M.M. (2002). Ruptured uterus eight year retrospective analysis of causes and management outcome in Adigrat Hospital, Tigray Region, Ethiopia. *Ethiopian Journal of Health Development*. 16(3), pp. 241-245.

6.Graham, S.B. (1991). When babies die: death and the education of obstetrical residents. *Medical Teacher*. 13(2), pp. 45-51.

7.Harden, R.M. (1996). Twelve tips on teaching and learning how to break bad news. *Medical Teacher*. 18(4), pp. 275-278.

8. Heazell,A. & McLaughlin,M.(2010) Stillbirth: Why did this happen? Midwives. February-March2010 pp. 46-47.

9. Hope, T; Savulescu, J; and Hendrick, J. (2004). *Medical Ethics and Law*. Edinburgh: Churchill Livingstone.

10. Hughes,P. The Management of Bereaved Mothers: What is Best? *Midwives Chronicle and Nursing Notes,* 1987; 8 : 226-236

11. Musters, C., McDonald, E. and Jones, I. (2008). Management of postnatal depression. *BMJ.* 337, pp. a736.

12. Ndosi, N.K, and Mtawali, M.L.W. (2002). The Nature of Puerperal Psychosis at Muhimbili National Hospital: Its Physical Co-Morbidity Associated Main Obstetric and Social Factors. *African Journal of Reproductive Health.* 6(1), pp. 41-49.

13. Murira, N. Communicating Sexual and Reproductive Health Messages: In search of a model to increase risk perception in primiparous women. PhD Thesis. 2010. Birmingham City University

14. Odusoga, O.L; Adefuye, P.O; Oloyede, O.A; Fakoya, T.A. and Olatunji, A.O. (2003). Uterine rupture: A major Contributor to Obstetric Morbidity in Sagamu. *Tropical Journal of Obstetrics and Gynaecology.* 20(2), pp. 137-140.

15. Reddy,U.M. (2007) Prediction and prevention of recurrent stillbirth. Obstet Gynecol 110(5) 1154-64

16. Tiegen, J. (2008) Parents needs for care and support when a child dies in stillbirth. International Stillbirth Conference, Oslo, Norway. International Stillbirth Alliance: Baltimore.

17. Weiss, G.L. and Larson, D.L. (1990). Health value, health locus of control, and the prediction of health protective behaviours. *Social Behaviour and Personality.* 18(1), pp. 121-135.

Chapter 8
IMMEDIATE BABY CARE

As soon as the baby is delivered, he must be assessed according to internationally accepted standards of well-being. This assessment is done at one minute and at ten minutes after delivery according to the Virginia Apgar Score as follows:

Fig. 8.1 The Apgar Score

Baby's Condition	0	1	2	1minute	5minutes	10minutes
Activity(muscle tone	Limp/Flaccid	Weak	Active			
Pulse/Heart rate	Absent	Bradycardia	Normal			
Response to stimuli Grimace, reflex, irritability	Absent	Weak	Active			
Appearance(skin colour)	Grey	Dusky	Pink			
Respiration	Absent	Rib recession/Gasping	Normal			
Total score						

The condition of the baby is scored on a ten point score. Each aspect is allocated two points. A score below five points at one minute of birth indicates that the baby is in danger and needs urgent assistance and close monitoring and expert care to improve the condition. Oxygen is given to improve the colour and breathing, and warmth is provided. The baby is expected to pick up points at the ten-minute assessment when usually the general condition improves.

Preventing Hypothermia

Soon after delivery, care should be taken to quickly wipe the baby and wrap the baby warmly in warm towels from head to toe in order to avoid loss of body heat before giving him to the mother. The baby's head should be thoroughly mopped dry to prevent hypothermia especially in cold months of the year and in those labour wards that are not well equipped to provide warmth when required. A heater may be made available to warm the air in the labour ward. Washing the baby immediately after delivery has no documented advantage and may predispose the baby to hypothermia.

Prevention of Bleeding

Babies are subjected to trauma and bruising during childbirth and may bleed post delivery. Close observation of the umbilical stump and the head is advised in order to identify incidence of bleeding early and take appropriate action such as additional clamping of the cord and administration of Vit. K.

Immediately after delivery, it is important to follow the agreed protocol on prevention and control of haemorrhage. Many labour wards' common practice is to give to the new born baby Vit.K1 intramuscularly to boost clotting factors and prevent haemorrhage.

Baby's Weight

The baby must be weighed immediately after delivery except where the baby's condition suggests otherwise such as where the baby requires immediate resuscitation or warmth of an incubator, then weighing can be delayed until the condition of the baby is favourable. Weighing the baby helps to assess if the baby's weight falls within the expected weight for gestation. This information forms essential baseline information that will be used for further management of the baby and to monitor baby's weight gain and developmental milestones. Most mothers take interest in the baby's birth weight and should be given this information soon after the baby is weighed.

Small for dates

A baby is small for gestation when his weight is below the expected percentile for the duration of pregnancy. A baby maybe born small for dates indicating some intra-uterine growth retardation. Babies likely to be born small are babies born to mothers with severe malnutrition before pregnancy, chronic diseases, infections such as malaria and poor circulation such as in hypertension and smoking in pregnancy (Morley,1979). Any conditions that interfere with circulation to the placenta may cause placental insufficiency resulting in fetal growth retardation. These conditions result in placental insufficiency or failure of the placenta to supply adequate nutrition to the baby. It is important to examine the placenta of infarcts which are patches of altered hard tissue suggesting poor circulation to the placenta and deterioration of the placenta. After the assessment of the baby, there should be close observation of the baby. The mother must be advised to keep the baby warm and feed the baby frequently. The baby must be weighed daily to observe weight changes.

Large for dates

A baby is large for dates when he weighs more that the average weight of babies born at a similar gestation. Babies may be large if born of big parents, if born of diabetic mother and where a mother had good nutrition. Babies born to diabetic mothers must be observed closely and blood sugar monitored.

Examination of the New Born Baby

The newborn baby must be examined from head to toe for congenital abnormalities and birth injuries immediately after delivery and before the baby is discharged home. The findings must be clearly recorded and taken note of as base line findings that can be referred to as the baby's growth and achievements are observed along the life span. The parents must be made aware of the findings and their importance. Should there be any findings to take note of, the parents should be fully informed of these and possible plan of action should be discussed with the parents.

Breathing

The baby is expected to expand the chest muscles and fill the lungs with air after a good cry at birth. Thereafter, the baby is expected to breathe smoothly and quietly. Babies move both the chest muscles and the abdominal muscles as they breathe. However a baby whose chest is sucked inwards, **rib recession,** as she breathes has difficulty in breathing. The airways must be cleared and oxygen must be administered to assist the baby to breathe smoothly. The baby must be transferred to an intensive care unit where possible. A baby who groans when breathing must be given oxygen. Difficulty in breathing may occur in premature babies, or may follow a difficult delivery, meconeum aspiration and fetal distress prior to delivery. In the case of meconeum aspiration, antibiotics must be administered.

The Skin Colour

The baby's skin must be observed for signs of *cyanosis.* A grey or dusky baby must be put on oxygen until the colour improves to a pink colour. The presence of fine hairs, *lanugo,* on the face may be an indication of prematurity. The baby must be managed as a premature baby until proved otherwise. Care must be taken to prevent the complications associated with prematurity.

Dry wrinkled skin is typical of post term babies. The greasy white substance that may coat the baby's skin at birth, *vernix carssiosa,* provides insulation to the baby while still in utero.

Birth marks, usually patches of darker or lighter skin than the rest of the body can be present. Birth marks are due to poor distribution of pigment.

Albinism

Some babies may be born with congenital absence of skin pigment, *albinism.* Some parents may feel ashamed and embarrassed to hold the baby in public. Some have felt cursed and wished the baby dead or adopted. Some mothers have been reported to refuse to feed the baby or refused to accept the baby as theirs.

Some families may engage in witch hunting and this may cause a lot of distress to the mother. Apart from reassurance, the baby's mother needs to be informed on how to keep the baby free from skin infections, and protecting the child from direct sun rays though the use of appropriate clothing and specific skin protection lotions. Parents are informed of the need for constant contact with the local health centre to keep the baby as healthy as possible. Advice on a good healthy diet should be provided. The parents should be reassured that albinos are intelligent and capable of a normal life like any other child. It is also important to inform the parents of special support clinics, clubs and associations for parents with children with similar problems.

The parents need to fully understand the nature of their child's problem in order to prepare them to look after the child in the best possible manner and to care for the child in the best possible manner.

The Head

Inspection and palpation of the head must be done to exclude haematoma and caput succedaneum. Caput succedaneum which is collection of serous fluid on the presenting part, may unduly lengthen the head. Cephalohaematoma, which is bleeding underneath the periosteum of the cranial bones is rarely identifiable immediately post delivery, but can be easily identified as swelling that does not cross a suture line 24 to forty eight hours post delivery. The shape of the head is greatly affected by the type of *moulding* that occurred during labour. Excessive moulding occurs especially in premature babies because the sutures are wide and the bones more pliable. Anencephaly is minimal development of the vault of the skull and the cerebral hemispheres of the brain. This abnormality is usually not compatible with life as the babies usually die immediately after delivery.

Hydrocephaly

The **sutures** must be gently traced using fingers to identify wide sutures which may be an indication of *prematurity* or. Where sutures are wide apart, the baby has to be closely monitored. The head circumference must be measured every day to check if it is increasing. The choroids plexus of the brain secrets cerebro-spinal fluid into the ventricles of the brain. This fluid ideally flows freely within the ventricles of the brain, the sub-arachnoid space of the spinal cord and washes the brain, keeping it moist. The venous sinuses in the brain continuously absorb the fluid. Obstruction of the sinuses results in accumulation of the cerebro-spinal fluid and dilation of the ventricles, resulting in development of hydrocephalus (Turner et al.,1988). The parents must be informed fully of the condition of the baby and the prognosis. They should be counselled and referred to a psychologist.

Microcephaly

Microcephaly is marked smallness of the skull. This is due to failure of the cerebral hemispheres of the brain to fully develop. The fontanelles may be closed or almost closed at birth. The head circumference should be measured with a tape measure at birth, and repeated at least forty-eight hours later when moulding and haematoma have subsided to exclude hydrocephalus and microcephally. The parents must be made fully aware of the condition and the likely developmental complications of the child. They should be advised to keep close observations of the baby and report to health personnel any complications arising.

The fontanelles

The fontanelles are wide areas of membranous tissue where two or more sutures meet. The fontanelles must be palpated. The anterior fontanel is found where the sagittal suture meets the two coronal sutures. The posterior fontanel is found where the sagittal suture and the lambdoidal sutures meet.In some babies, the posterior fontanel may not be palpable and almost closed especially in post term babies, while in others it may be palpable. .

The Eyes

The eyes are not easy to open and examine immediately after delivery. The size of the eyes must be equal and the eyes well set. It maybe too early and difficult to detect signs of **strabismus** or determine whether the baby has eyesight or is blind. However vision is present but limited. Babies are known to see images and bright light. Baby's eye reactions that early may be sluggish.

Tears from the eyes could be an indication of blockage of the lachrymal ducts or irritation due to bruises during birth. Indurations too follow strain during delivery. Most of it clears within 48 hours. The baby must be closely observed for further haemorrhage. Eye discharge may not be apparent immediately after delivery but it is advisable to start treating babies born of mothers with sexually transmitted diseases immediately post delivery.

Ears

Lowly set ears may be a sign of trisomy 21. Accessory auricles may be found on the front of the ears. Accessory auricles can be ligated and allowed to dry and drop off. Where there is doubt on what action to take, the baby must be referred to a paediatrician as soon as possible.

The Nose

Patency of both nostrils must be tested. A suction catheter inserted in the nostrils to clear the airways is an effective test for patency of the nostrils. In -drawing of the nostrils as the baby breathes, and mouth breathing could be signs of upper respiratory tract blockage, *choanal atresia.*

Froth from the nostrils and cyanosis may be suggestive of *tracheo-oesophageal fistula,* a common opening between the oesophagus and the trachea. It is important to refer the baby immediately for assessment by a paediatrician. It is advisable to withhold feeding the baby orally until confirmation from the paediatrician is obtained. Parents must be informed about the condition of their baby and the possible management of the condition. Parents will have a lot of questions to ask and factual responses must be provided.

The Mouth

The lips must be inspected for *harelip.* The hard and soft palate must be inspected for *cleft palate*, which may be complete to extend to the nostrils. It may be unilateral or bilateral as a result of failure of the palatine bones to fuse. Cleft palate may be present on its on or the baby may have a hare-lip as well.

Parents of babies with cleft palate need a lot of psychological support as well as skills to master how to feed the baby before leaving hospital and need reassurance that the baby's mouth can be successfully repaired. Parents must be informed about the availability of special feeding teats and use of a spoon in feeding the baby. It is best for the parents to leave the hospital with a date for the repair of the abnormality known in order to lessen the depression and give them hope. The relatives have to be counselled as well. Regular postnatal follow up should be made to provide the much needed psychological and skills support.

Gum Cysts

The mouth is examined for gum cysts, and any other abnormalities. Gum cysts may appear like early signs of teething and may cause undue anxiety in new parents and some cultures Gum cysts burst on their own as the baby begins to move his jaws vigorously when breast feeding. Some babies may be born with one or two teeth. They can be referred to the dentist.

The Tongue

The size of the tongue must be observed. A large tongue, macroglossia, that fills the mouth and sticks out, *glossoptosis,* is associated with trisomal defects like **Down's Syndrome/Trisomy 21** A new born with this type of congenital abnormality has some of the following features:

- Low birth weight.
- A short antero-posterior diameter of the head, making the head smaller than is expected, (microcephaly)
- The baby has a flat face, a small nose,
- Protruding tongue, glossoptosis
- The eyes may be poorly focused.
- The ears are lowly set and the ear folds are poorly developed.
- The hands are flat with a single palmer crease across the palms and short, inward curved little fingers, *clinodactyly.*
- The feet are flat and have a wide gap between the large toe and second toe (Turner et al.,1988).

It is important that a paediatrician confirms the diagnosis.

The parents must be supported psychologically and information on the condition and other support services available provided. A baby with Down's syndrome can shock a primiparous mother and may lead to varying degrees of depression.

Critical incident

> Miss Ellen a 39year old banker delivered her first baby girl with marked vivid features of Down's syndrome. She was visited by a health visitor two days after discharge from hospital. Miss Ellen's face was swollen showing that she had been crying. She broke down when the health visitor asked her how she and the baby were."Why me? Why should I get this? Look at me, I own this bungalow, I have everything I need. I have a good job and I felt it was time I had a child, and this is what I get?"
>
> She could not bear put the baby to breast. "I can't hold it let alone 'put it' onto my breast!' She sobbed uncontrollably. 'I have asked my friends not to visit. I will give people something to talk about. I can't keep it!"(Murira,2010)

After a lot of persuasion, Miss Ellen was persuaded to feed the baby artificially while a social worker made arrangements to take the baby into a children's home. Miss Ellen needed the services of a psychologist and a counsellor thereafter. It cannot be overemphasized that women need professional support in their homes especially in the first week after delivery.

Oesophageal Atresia

Excessive salivation and mucus is suggestive of blockage of the upper oesophagus, *oesophageal atresia.* A naso-gastric tube that fails to go down the gastro-intestinal tract could be suggestive of this condition. The baby should be referred to the paediatrician immediately for further management. The baby's parents must be informed of the need for the paediatrician to examine the baby without unduly raising the anxiety levels or causing fear in them.

The Jaws

The cheekbones should be proportional to the size of face. Mandibular hypoplasia, *micrognathia,* or small mandible can be present. This is referred to as the *Pierre-Robin Syndrome*. The baby may feed slowly requiring extreme patience during feeding. It is important to expose the parents to as much information as possible about the condition, reassure them and give them as much support as possible.

The Chest

Swollen Breast/s

One or both breasts of the baby may be swollen due to the effect of withdrawal of maternal oestrogen. Mothers should be reassured that the swelling will subside without need for treatment.

The Abdomen

Baby's abdomen is proportionally larger than the chest. Too large an abdomen may be an indication of internal bleeding. Imperfect closure of the abdominal wall may result in umbilical *hernia*, abdominal contents protruding below the skin around the umbilicus and *exomphallus,* the entire abdominal contents outside the abdominal wall. The bladder may be outside the abdominal wall, *ectopia vesicae.* Such abnormalities should be quickly referred to surgeons for correction.

The umbilical stump is checked for bleeding with each nappy change. It may be necessary to apply two cord clamps where the umbilical stump is thick to secure it and prevent bleeding.

The Skeletal System

The size of limbs and bones must be proportional to the size of the body. In *achondroplasia*, the limbs are relatively short compared to the other parts of the body. The head is larger than the rest of the body structures. The parents of such a baby must be reassured as such babies usually develop normally mentally and are capable of learning and developing into independent individuals.

The Back

The baby is turned round and the back is examined. **Scoliosis**, a deformity of the vertebral column where usually the thoracic vertebral column curves abnormally, may be present.

Spina Bifida, a defect in the closure of the spinal cord and commonly found in the lumbar-sacral region may be present. The contents of the cord may be visible and herniated through the defect. Sometimes the meninges only protrude out, in which case the deformity is called a *meningocele.*

When the meninges together with nerve tissue are part of the hernia, the deformity is called **myelomeningocele.** This may present as a raw fleshy area or a hairy mole. The deformity is corrected surgically. The parents of such a baby need a lot of emotional support. It is best that surgical correction is done before the baby is taken home to prevent infection.

The Hands

The arms must be the same length. Movement of the arms must be equal. A baby who does not freely move one arm could have a birth injury such as a fracture or dislocation. Such injuries should be looked out for especially after difficult breech delivery or in big babies where shoulder dystocia could have occurred. Arrangements must be made to have an x-ray of the passive arm to exclude fractures.

Extra digits are among the commonest minor congenital abnormality found on new born babies. If the extra digit is attached by skin, which is commonly the case, the extra digit is tightly tied with silk where it is joined to the main finger or toe. It should fall off within the first week. It may be necessary to review the knot, which may loosen up before the skin dries off. A fresh knot is applied to allow the skin to shrivel. If the digit is joined by bone, then the advice of the orthopaedic surgeon should be sought. The parents must always be reassured and the nature of intervention explained clearly.

The Legs

The legs should be equal in length and equally active. Signs of fractures and dislocation of the hips especially after difficult breech delivery must be excluded. *Osteogenesis Imperfecta* or brittle bones should be looked out for. The little feet must be examined for *tallipes and clubfoot,* and if present, the baby must be referred immediately for surgical attention. Parents are distraught by congenital abnormalities and health personnel must communicate with the parents responding to their questions with factual responses.

The Genitals

Some baby features which may worry new mothers are male babies may be born with the urethral opening on the under surface of the penis, *hypospadiasis*. Mothers should be reassured about this feature, which usually corrects itself as the baby grows older. Extensive deformities may be corrected surgically.

The size of the scrotal sac is determined by the presence or absence of the testes in the scrotal sac. It should be remembered that testes move back and forth into the abdomen through the inguinal canal until this structure narrows with growth. Mothers should be reassured about this. *Undescended testes* may however remain in the inguinal canal or become obstructed resulting in a hernia

Vulval Bleed/Discharge

Female babies may have a mucoid, milky or bloody discharge from the vulva. Mothers should be reassured that the mucoid and milky discharge is normal. The bloody discharge, which is the result of the influence of the withdrawal of maternal female hormones, should clear away within a few days.

Patency of the anal and urethral orifices

Some babies readily pass meconeum during or immediately after delivery. When exposed to the room temperature after delivery, most babies empty their bladders. Where the bowels have not opened, a thermometer is passed as if to take the rectal temperature in order to check for the rectal patency. To check for urethral patency, the mother is advised to report as soon as the baby wets his nappy.

All abnormalities identified must be noted and clearly written in the baby' notes.

Parental Support

The parents of the newborn must be informed of any abnormality identified on the baby. Abnormalities in the newborn may frustrate a young mother to the point of severe depression. Whenever a woman delivers a baby with a **cleft palate, exomphalus, spina bifida, hydrocephalic** and other gross abnormalities, the looks of the baby may scare a young mother to depression. Such mothers and their spouses need counselling and a one to one client education to help them understand fully the condition of the baby, the likely management and how to cope with the baby on a day-to-day basis. The spouses must be involved in the counselling. They must be informed of the implications of the abnormality and the likely course of care. Parents will need as much information as possible on the abnormality to help them look after the baby in the best way possible. Parents need to know what to expect as the child grows so that they can make informed decisions about the child's health and be able to identify good progress, or retardation and to be able to report these.

Specialist paediatricians must be consulted for advice on further management of the infant. Parents are naturally shocked to see abnormalities on their babies and will need repeated counselling to accept the baby. However it is not all parents who will be prepared to look after a baby with a congenital abnormality. Some parents may want to surrender the baby to an institution. It is important that parents are given as much information as possible on availability of such institutions. The parents of babies with congenital abnormalities considered genetic will need genetic counselling and should be informed of available tests, specialists and any corrective measures available.

Checking for Reflexes

The baby's reaction to various tests must be checked to assess for alertness and normalcy in the baby.

The Rooting Reflex

This is testing for the baby's reaction to suckling reflexes. A finger gently moved on the cheeks from the angles of the mouth should make the baby turn his head towards the finger and make sucking movements. Placing baby onto the mother's chest, immediately after delivery, however best tests the sucking reflex. The baby should be able to find the breast and start suckling. Alternatively, where the baby is alert, he can be applied to the mother's breast and should be able to start suckling immediately.

The Walking /Stepping Reflex

When baby is put on his feet, he attempts to lift his foot to walk. Failure to lift legs shows weakness and probable injury of the nerves of the legs which is more likely in difficult breech delivery.

Moro Reflex

When a baby is suddenly lowered down, he panics, and suddenly extends and abducts his limbs. Birth injuries involving nerves may be identified by observing the reaction of the limbs.

The Grasp Reflex

If a finger is placed in the newborn's hand, the baby grasps the finger tightly so much that it is possible to test for traction and muscle tone. Weak grasp or failure to grasp the finger is an indication of weakness mostly due to injury of the radial or ulna nerves. The baby must be referred to neuro- specialists.

Asymmetrical Tonic Neck Reflex

When the baby's neck is passively turned to the side, the limbs on the same side to which the neck is turned are extended while those on the opposite side are flexed. This is suggestive of neck injury at birth especially after breech delivery and shoulder dystocia.

Glabellar Reflex

When the root or the nose is gently tapped, the eyes are screwed.

The responsiveness of the baby to the reflexes is an indication of the alertness or passivity of the baby.

N.B. A baby, who has been subjected to a difficult labour, or needed resuscitation of one type or another, may not have positive reflexes immediately after delivery. It is advisable to repeat the test for reflexes after twenty- four hours to forty-eight hours to give the baby an opportunity to recover from the stress of labour. If however the absence of reflexes persists, the baby must be referred to a specialist neurologist.

Soon after examination, the baby must be warmly wrapped to avoid *hypothermia neonatorum.* Where the spouse is available, it is very important to involve him by giving him a chance to participate in the activities going on by holding the baby after the examination is done, and allowing him space close to his partner. It is important to give the couple a chance to be on their own with their baby.

Congenital Syphilis

 Syphilis is transmitted from the mother to the fetus via the placenta after sixteen weeks gestation when the placenta is fully developed. Congenital syphilis is preventable and occurs only where the pregnant women and their partners are not treated. The more recent infection in the mother the higher the risk of the baby contracting the disease. Skin lesions are present on the fetus at birth. *Bullous eruptions* in the palms and soles of feet, the groins and popular lesions of the nose and mouth can be seen. The infant has a typical *saddle nose* discharging muco-purulent or blood stained discharge that causes snuffles and difficulty in feeding. A typical *old man's look* with fissures around the mouth can be seen on the face. A generalized *lymphadenopathy* is present. *The liver* and *spleen* are enlarged. The infant may have *hydrocephalus.* The baby must be referred to a paediatrician immediately. The parents are counselled and commenced on treatment.

A postnatal leaflet that discusses essentials of baby care should be made available to mothers on leaving hospital.

Care for the newborn is a full time job and a few new mothers may not be prepared for that. Advice on sharing love and involving the spouse in looking after the baby, and sharing care of the baby in such chores as bathing the baby, clothing the baby including changing the nappies should be encouraged and should be part of parenthood preparation for both parents.

References

1. Turner,TL; Douglas,J; Corkburn,F. Craig's Care of the Newly Born Infant. 8th Ed.Churchill Livingstone, 1988.
2. Morley,D. Paediatric Priorities in the Developing World. Butterworths. 1979

Chapter 9

BABY FEEDING

Each baby is a unique individual and should be treated as such. Some babies are ready to latch onto the breast immediately they are close to the mother's breast. Other babies, especially those that have endured a long difficult labour and have needed resuscitation may be too tired to suckle immediately. The closeness to the mother maybe all that the baby requires for a while. Some mothers too may be too tired to be enthusiastic to breast-feed immediately. Each woman and each baby must be managed according to their condition post delivery and not according to routine protocols.

Free flow of milk is not until the third day after delivery. Many women are worried that their babies will starve without adequate milk in the first two or three days before full establishment of the milk flow. It is the duty of the midwives to explain to the mothers about the rich composition of colostrum and how it satisfies the baby needs and its laxative element that enables the baby to empty its bowel of meconeum.

Breast-Feeding

'Mother' means one who nurtures. Nurturing or tendering is believed to be enabled by successful breast feeding. Breast feeding is exclusive for most African women and especially for the Shona women of Zimbabwe is the expected cultural norm. The baby must not be allowed to starve. The women's mentors emphasize the mother's role as that of breast-feeding her newborn baby. Women who fail to breast feed successfully are considered a disgrace as they are unable to achieve goals of womanhood. The first three days post delivery are therefore critical in a young woman who must master the skills of successful breast-feeding. A new mother is expected to effectively care for her delicate baby, and grasp the relevant skills to apply the baby to the breast and to enable the baby to suckle successfully. The female culture expects women to breast feed their babies until the baby can talk and can demand to be breast fed. Inability to achieve this culturally expected and accepted maternal function suggests that a young primiparous woman needs not only information support but also needs practical support post delivery.

Some problems that may contribute to poor baby feeding such as cracked nipples, flat nipples or failure to breast feed because the baby's suckling hurt, have been observed in primiparous women.

Physiologically breast feeding increases blood oxytocin levels and may prevent menses in some breast feeding women decreasing the threat of another pregnancy too soon. Breast feeding is thought culturally to inform the body to *wait till the nurturing function of the woman's body is complete*. Breastfeeding is considered by the Shona female culture as one way of taking control of the body system is believed to have two functions, that of nurturing and that of controlling the natural physiological event of conception.

Successful breast-feeding is one of the major goals of the postnatal period (Hofvander, 2005). Some cultures are reported to stop breast feeding as soon as they have minor problems such as sore nipples and poor latching on the breast. Sometimes breast feeding is stopped to enable the partner to participate in baby feeding (Hunter, 2008). Shona women, on the contrary, do not expect their partners to have an active role to play soon after the baby is born and men have limited contact with the baby. The lack of partner involvement in the immediate puerperium is an accepted practice in the particular culture. This controlled contact with one's spouse is considered necessary to allow for the cultural rituals to be completed before the couple lives together after the birth of a child. This practice has its shortfalls especially that successful parenting starts with early bonding between father and the newborn child.

In the first three days post delivery, naturally lactation is not fully established for most women but the breasts have the rich nutritious *colostrum* that the baby can feed on. In the Shona culture, elderly women are not satisfied that there is adequate milk in the breast until they see a steady flow of milk when the breast is expressed. Elderly women believe that the breasts need stimulation and must be 'awakened' to start functioning to effect lactation. The elderly women may respond to the slow establishment of lactation in the new mother by making incisions into the breast tissue of the young women with a razor blade and filling up the incisions with ground ash of burnt leaves from a specific shrub, believed to be a 'lactation stimulant.' This practice has been observed to be wide spread and the explanation is the same suggesting that this is a widely accepted practice (Murira,2010). Within these first few days before lactation is established, there may be efforts to give the baby varied preparations from water, oil, thin porridge, fruit juice, glucose and artificial powdered milks, cow's milk, goat's milk, camel's milk and many other preparations. The older women are only too happy to offer explanations of beliefs, taboos and practices to justify the observed practices.

Ideally, the young primiparous women need continuous support post delivery until they are confident to feed the baby successfully. The exposure of the young women to potentially dangerous practices can only justify and emphasize the need for health information on physiology of puerperium and lactation and continuous health professionals' support of the new mother. The physiology of lactation must be explained to new mothers in simple language, so that they do not resort to dangerous practices that may cause constipation, indigestion and malnutrition to the baby. It is also possible to introduce into the mother, infections such as mastitis and breast abscess, in some of the attempts to improve lactation

The wide spread engagement in ineffective and potentially dangerous cultural practices can be translated to be indicators that women need effective post natal self-care skills. Women need information to empower them in risk prevention especially to enable them to differentiate safe from potentially dangerous practices post delivery.

Studies in other cultures have revealed varied cultural practices around the post natal period in which women have a set of traditional behaviors to follow post delivery, some of which are detrimental to the women's health. Suggestions have been made to assess the impact of cultural practices on the women's health to assist in the designing of appropriate health education and health promotion programmes (Kaewsarm et al., 2003; Wang et al., (2008).

Women should be encouraged to give their babies human milk specifically prepared for human consumption unless there are special contraindications to feeding the baby on human milk. The midwife should explain to the mothers in laymen's language the advantages of breast milk and breast feeding.

Breast Feeding advantages

Breast milk is the natural baby's milk, and contains immune bodies to prevent infections in the baby

Breast milk is available all the time. The mother must be encouraged to drink fluids to encourage an increased flow.

Breast milk is always at the right temperature so it does not need warming

Breast milk is nutritious with all food values in the correct proportions

Breast milk is whole; there is no need for additives

Breast milk is environment friendly, it does not create litter in its production and after use

Breast milk is easily stored and cannot be contaminated by dust or any environmental wastes as it is within the mother

Breast milk is economical, there are no expenses incurred to acquire it

Breast milk promotes close relationships between mother and baby

The importance of a nutritious diet and taking plenty of fluids to improve the flow of milk should be emphasized.

Common Positions For Breast Feeding

The positions a mother can adapt to breast feed her baby are many depending on whether she is seated or lying in bed. Post delivery abdominal muscles may still be overstretched in such a way that some new mothers may have the problems of successfully applying their babies to the breast. A pillow or cushion placed under the baby's shoulders will help the baby reach the breast with relative ease.

The baby can lie across the lap supported by one arm, while the other arm directs the breast into the baby's mouth. This is the most common position adopted by many women. A baby may be placed under the arm with legs freely moving. This is most comfortable for mothers who have had a caesarean section whose abdomens are tender and the baby's activity may cause some discomfort. The mother holds the back of the bead and supports baby's shoulders with her forearm. The baby reaches the breast fairly easily in this position.

Sitting the baby on the lap facing the breast, the forearm supports baby's trunk, while the palm and fingers support the head. The baby is close to the breast. This is especially suitable for the nulliparous mother whose breasts are still erect and do not necessarily *fall* into the baby's mouth.

While the mother is lying on her side, breast-feeding can successfully be carried out. This position is convenient where the mother feels tired, or less confident to hold the baby to the breast or more comfortable in a lying position. After perineal repair many mothers may find this position most convenient. The mother lies on her side facing her baby and directs the breast into the baby's mouth while one hand cuddles the baby. Some mothers may find it easy to prop the baby on the forearm to enable baby to reach the breast. Many babies enjoy this position and may latch onto the breast for long periods especially at night. Mothers must be advised to ensure that baby's nostrils are clear of the breast.

N.B. It is advisable that the mother is awake as she breast feeds to ensure that she observes the baby as he feeds.

Observation during feeding

The mother is advised to keep her eyes on the baby when breast-feeding in case the breasts block the baby's nostrils during feeding. Blocking the baby's nostrils is prevented by holding the breast with four fingers under the breast and the thumb retracting excess breast folds from the baby's nostrils. The baby may vomit and choke or inhale vomitus. During feeding, observing baby's colour helps to identify early signs of choking. Baby's colour must always remain pink. If the baby should look greyish in colour when feeding, this suggests blockage of airways. Feeding must be stopped immediately to allow the baby to breath freely and to investigate the cause of change of colour in the baby.

The baby is best put to sleep on his side after a feed. This prevents possible accidents of choking and inhaling the vomitus should the baby regurgitate the feed. Should the baby regurgitate while he lies on his side, the regurgitated feed will flow onto the side away from baby's nostrils.

Winding/Burping

Burping the baby when he looks satisfied ensures that he lets out wind that he unintentionally swallows as he feeds. This also ensures that the baby is observed as he lets out wind in case he brings up the feed and chokes on it. Burping ensures that baby does not get colicky pain which may be uncomfortable that baby cries continuously. Some mothers may quickly resort to expensive off the counter medication to relieve their babies of this wind the baby swallows during feeding. Mothers should be taught how to burp their babies to relieve them of the wind.

Assisting Baby to Burp

The baby can be held against the parent's chest with the head supported by the parent's shoulder. One arm supports the baby while the other arm gently pats the baby's back until the baby belches.

The baby may be put across the parent's lap. One arm can support the baby's head and neck while the other pats or caresses the baby's back.

If a mother is confident, she can sit the baby on her lap and supports the baby with one arm while the other caresses the baby's back until the baby belches.

After the baby lets out wind, he should be allowed to feed again as he will have created some space.

Mothers should be informed that a baby who does not seem to settle is likely to be hungry. Mothers are encouraged to keep the baby on the breast for long periods to ensure that the baby has enough milk.

Problems in Breast Feeding

Poor Lactation

A new mother may feel discouraged by what may seem to be poor milk flow and may easily be tempted to look for alternative ways of baby feeding. Many mothers think that they do not produce adequate amounts of milk when their problem is inadequate intake of fluids. Before any alternatives are sought, it is important to ensure that the mother takes plenty of oral fluids to improve lactation, fruit juices and fortified milk drinks must be encouraged. Fizzy drinks and any drinks with high levels of alcohol should be discouraged.

Mothers with small breasts must be reassured that even the small breasts can produce adequate amounts of milk to satisfy a baby's needs.

The Baby's feeding needs

Some mothers may feel that the baby needs more milk than their breasts are capable of producing and may want to supplement the breast milk. A baby that cries a few minutes after feeding, a baby who hangs onto the breast and continues to suckle, a baby whose skin remains wrinkled and rough, and has a sunken fontanel, a baby who passes little or concentrated urine that stains the nappy after a long while, and a baby who seems restless and frantic and opens his mouth making sucking movements or sounds, is sending a message that the milk intake is inadequate.

A satisfied baby sleeps for long periods. A well -hydrated baby passes clear urine frequently.

Flat Nipples

Some primiparous mothers may have problems fixing the baby onto the breast especially where the nipple is not raised enough above the surface of the breast making it difficult for the baby to latch successfully during feeding. A mother with this problem may be advised to continue to put baby to breast until the nipple shapes up. It maybe necessary to use a breast pump where it is available to help the nipple to protrude out. A breast pump will serve two purposes, that of expressing milk, which can later be used to feed the baby and also pulling the nipple forward to prominence.

Where a breast pump is not available, a mother can be advised to hold the nipple between the index finger and the thumb and roll it gently for a while especially during bath times. The nipple will with time take shape.

Cracked Nipples

Successful breast-feeding occurs when the baby's lips firmly grip the areola of the breast while the nipple is held between the baby's palate and the tongue as the baby suckles. Failure to achieve this position results in the baby sucking in the nipple whose thin skin quickly gives way. The baby is not usually satisfied in such a situation and may hang onto the breast for long periods further complicating the situation. The baby may cry immediately after feeding indicating that he is not satisfied.

Home remedies such as applying petroleum jelly to the nipple should be discouraged as the baby may be put off the breast by the taste of the petroleum jelly. This practice causes further cracking of nipples as damage to the nipple may occur while trying to wipe off the petroleum jelly. Where nipples are dry the mother should be encouraged to use her milk to soften the nipple by first expressing a little milk then gently spread it on the nipple and areola. After feeding the baby the *"hind" milk,* which is thicker and richer can be applied on the nipple and areola and the nipple will heal naturally. The mother should be taught how to properly 'fix' the baby on the breast.

Bruised or cracked nipples are very painful that an inexperienced mother may be tempted to put the baby off that breast temporarily resulting in another problem, that of engorgement

Breast Complications

Mastitis

Two cultural practices have been observed to exacerbate breast complications and these are the 'lactation stimulants' which result in women developing mastitis within 24hours of the breast incisions. After lactation is fully established the women suffer from engorged breasts and the elderly women attribute the full breasts to the success of herbal treatment of the breasts. Many young women fail to apply their babies to the breast successfully thereafter because of the inflammation. The tender and painful breasts may suppurate causing breast abscesses that require incision and drainage resulting in protracted breast feeding problems (Murira, 2010).

The second practice that has been observed is as a result of a belief that if the baby belches on the breast during breast feeding, the milk in the particular breast is thought to be poisonous for at least twenty-four hours. The affected breast naturally over- fills and becomes swollen and very uncomfortable for the young woman. These lactation beliefs may expose young women to severe pain and discomfort post delivery. Failure to breast feed compounds the socio-economic problems of women especially from a low social economic background as they may not afford commercial baby products and alternative means to feed their babies. This situation impacts negatively on the health of both the babies and their mothers.

Engorged Breasts

Mothers should be alerted of the dangers of prevalent traditional practices and must be reassured of the safety of their milk even after the baby belches on the breast. As baby suckles, he draws in air which accumulates in the stomach. It is the presence of these air bubbles that causes the belching even in the middle of a feed. The breast-feeding mother must be informed that belching does not affect the breast milk in any way. In the event of breast engorgement, the breast-feeding mother is advised to feed the baby from the engorged breast first before feeding on the soft breast to relieve the engorgement. With the next feed, the baby should be put to the breast he last fed on during the previous feeding time. Alternating breasts at baby feeding times ensures that each breast has an equal chance of being emptied relieving the overfilling.

When the baby fails to empty the breasts completely a feeding mother is advised to express the milk and prevent the discomfort of an engorged breast. Manual expression can be done or a breast pump can be used. Avoiding cracks on nipples and ensuring that the breasts are emptied whenever baby is satisfied can prevent breast engorgement. Excess milk can be expressed and thrown away or refrigerated for baby's next feed.

Dribbling of breast milk through the mother's clothes can be very unsightly and embarrassing at times. Mothers can be advised to pad their breasts to avoid the dribbling. A large firm brassiere with wide straps to accommodate the filling breasts and hold them comfortably is advisable. Where women can afford they can be informed on the use of a feeding brassiere especially designed for breast-feeding mothers.

Breast Abscess

If an engorged breast is not emptied, an abscess may form. This may require incision and drainage and treatment with antibiotics. It may result in the baby having to feed from one breast for the time the affected breast is under treatment.

Artificial Feeding

Unlike the previous school of thought that prescribed breast-feeding on mothers, the progressive thought respects the wishes of individuals and their freedom of choice to bring up their children the way they feel is comfortable for them. Some parents may decide not to breast feed for cosmetic reasons. Some women may feel because of their demanding careers they may not afford adequate time to breast-feed. Some may have underlying conditions that makes breast feeding contraindicated maybe because of the nature of the conditions or because of the medication they may be on. Some of these conditions are HIV and AIDS, Tuberculosis, Cancer, heart disease and any such disease that would make breast feeding a strain on the mother.

Parents of multiple births have a genuine need to supplement the breast milk. Many working mothers leave their babies under the care of baby minders and may combine both breast and artificial feeding or wean their babies completely off the breast. These are realities in baby care that health personnel must be prepared to meet.

If a mother chooses to feed her baby artificially, the health personnel's role is to ensure that the mother has the skills to hygienically prepare the feeds and sterilise the utensils.

Mothers should be advised to closely observe their babies before leaving a health institution in order to pick out some of the obvious abnormalities and report back as quickly as they notice anything suspect on the baby.

Client Education

Each client must be offered **personalised education** that pertains to her health needs(Glaister & Michael,2006). Health personnel should identify **the teachable moments** and capitalise on them to offer pertinent information about the mother and her baby during this contact with health personnel(Lawson & Flowke,2008). Clients value the information given to them individually and feel obliged to comply with it because it is directed to them. Women need information on the likely post natal discomforts, diet that promotes quick healing of wounds and promotes good lactation, relationships with partner, suitable family planning methods, suitable exercises post delivery, and information on subsequent pregnancies.

Patient education is best given when a client is as comfortable as possible (Ley,1988). Hurried large group education efforts when clients are ready to leave hospital may not be as effective as individualised information. A client uncomfortably seated due to a painful episiotomy wound, or worried about how she will get home, is unlikely to listen and assimilate health information. There is not enough time to give all the mothers the attention they deserve in the last minutes before they leave the hospital. Time should be created while the client is still in hospital to teach new mothers basic skills in baby and self care and to test the mother's competence in these skills. Such skills like putting baby to the breast, burping the baby, changing nappies, cleaning the umbilicus, bathing the baby, are some of the skills that mothers must master before leaving hospital.

References

1. Epstein, R.M. (2006). Making communication research matter: What do patients notice, what do patients want, and what do patients need? *Patient Education and Counselling.* 60, pp. 272-278.

2. Glaister, K. and Michael, M. (2006). Patient Health Education Literature. *International Journal of Health Promotion and Education.* 44(2), pp. 83-88.

3. Hofvander, Y. (2005). Breastfeeding and the Baby Friendly Hospitals Initiative: organization, response and outcome in Sweden and other countries. *Acta Paediatrica.* 94(8), pp. 1012-1016.

4. Hunter, L. (2008). Teenagers' experiences of postnatal care and breastfeeding. *British Journal of Midwifery.* 16(12), pp. 785-790.

5. Kaewsarn, P., Moyle, W. and Creedy, D. (2003). Traditional postpartum practices among Thai women. *Journal of Advanced Nursing.* 41(4), pp. 358-366.

6. Lawson, P.J. and Flocke, S.A. (2009). Teachable moments for health behaviour change: A concept analysis. *Patient Education and Counseling.* 76(1), pp. 25-30.

7. Ley, P. (1988). *Communicating with Patients: Improving Communication, Satisfaction, and Compliance.* London: Croom Helm.

8. Murira,N.Communicating sexual and reproductive health messages. In search of a model to increase risk perception among primiparous women.PhD Thesis.2010 Birmingham City University.

9. Wang, X., Wang, Y., Zanzhou, S., Wang, J. and Wang, J. (2008). A population based survey of women's traditional postpartum behaviours in Northern China. *Midwifery*. 24(2), pp. 238-245.

Chapter 10

EMPOWERING THE POSTNATAL MOTHER

Many postnatal mothers are poorly informed of their rights as consumers of health care services. Although health care is a commodity, which should be available to everyone, it is not readily available or advertised on the market like other commodities people need on a day-to-day basis. Information about available services needs to be passed on to the mothers to enable them to decide on whether they need the service or not. Health personnel or medical insurances should leave that decision to use a service to the health care client.

Women must be assisted to achieve control of their health in order for them to have full participation in their own health. Women's health education should include empowering women with inquisitive skills and assertiveness in issues of direct concern to them such as access to services of their choice like post natal care so that decision making in their health is transferred from members of the health team to the women themselves. Women should be assisted to access any service of their choice as and when they see fit.

The need for a post natal service should be much higher in the third world where basic information on self care is not readily available and women leave health care

Institutions early before they are exposed to any care skills.

Constant evaluation of how well the health sector is bringing health to the people and whether the health sector is achieving the objectives should be continuously evaluated. It is also important to establish if women's health needs are being addressed holistically. A strong well-structured continuous community care programme with a multi-professional team approach ensures that women are constantly in touch with health care services and can access information which empowers them to make informed health decisions.

Transferring skills to clients should be possible if client education is an inaugural part of client care.

Women's health information expressed in simple everyday languages to suit the varied clientele is essential throughout the child bearing period. Post delivery women need information to participate meaningfully in their care and the care of their new born infants. Step by step written information on procedures like baby bath, umbilical toilet, or fixing the baby to the breast should be made available to women on leaving health institutions post delivery. Where the level of literacy is low, pictorial leaflets could be used.

Health personnel working in a particular area, should develop a culture of writing leaflets, booklets and books that are culture sensitive and meeting the level of literacy for their clientele. Information heard is easily distorted and forgotten, whereas written literature can always be revisited, and passed on to other women. Client education should be the mainstay of the contact with a client and every teachable moment should be capitalized upon.

There should be a deliberate effort to move away from risk factor identification and management of ill health to "an orientation towards wellness" in which the mother is empowered to take charge of her health through making available relevant information she may need. The amount of time spent with each client is dependant on her health information needs and the need for specific skills as identified in the process of assessment and examination. Some mothers may therefore need more attention than others.

Critical incident

Mrs. Ushe delivered her first child by vaginal delivery but had to have a vacuum extraction for poor maternal effort. When she left hospital she and the baby seemed well. Forty- eight hours later, her baby started twitching on one side of the body. Her mother-in -law noticed that the baby had a red ring deeply marked on the head. The baby's head looked deformed around the ring. Mrs Ushe did not understand what was happening to the baby. This was reported to Mr. Ushe who concluded that Mrs. Ushe had carelessly dropped the baby on its head. When the health visitor arrived for a home visit, Mrs. Ushe was nursing a swollen black eye after being assaulted by her husband. She was so distressed that she had decided to leave her husband. Her in-laws present were not sympathetic with her.

Although the midwife provided an explanation when she arrived on a post natal visit, the incident had already damaged Mrs Ushe's relationship with her husband and in-laws.

The above incident could have been avoided had health personnel taken time to inform Mrs. Ushe about complications that are associated with instrumental deliveries.

Babies delivered with the assistance of a vacuum extractor and forceps may show complications after they have long left hospital. Facial palsy, twitching of facial muscles, induration of eyes, have been reported and observed in babies assisted by forceps at delivery, while haematoma on the head, fits, palsies and alopecia have been reported and observed in babies assisted by vacuum extraction.

Who Primiparous Mothers Live With Post Delivery

More than half of primiparous women preferred to live with their mothers, followed sisters, then husbands, then grandmothers post delivery in that order.

The reasons behind these choices are, that older women have experience in baby care and can help with the baby at night. Women who choose to live with their spouses may have a mother moving in with them and do so where health facilities are a distant away and spouses have means of transport. Murira (2010)'s personal observations of the Shona women and their newborn infants in the postnatal period revealed prevalent traditional cultural beliefs, values and practices.

Baby Care Practices

Baby care is an important aspect of post natal care. Babies need easy access to their mothers for love, cuddling and stimulation, appropriate feeding, appropriate environmental temperature, a safe environment that protects them from disease, harmful practices and abuse, cleanliness and an informed source to observe for signs of ill health and provision of appropriate health care (WHO, 2004). There are life-threatening illnesses that occur in the first week of birth resulting in death of infants and certain cultural practices that compromise the health of newborn babies (WHO,2004; Thompson,2003).

Women who stayed with elderly members of their families post delivery, used "herbal" treatments for various reasons on their babies (Murira,2003).

Neonatal Problems

Congenital abnormalities such as development of hydrocephalus, cleft palate, hair lip and Down's syndrome have been observed to disturb parents who cannot come to terms with the unfamiliar features. The use of herbal "treatments" on babies among the Shona was rampant especially in women who chose to live with elderly family women. Some babies were lost through ingestion of strong herbal preparations thought to promote good health and protect babies against evil spirits. The effect of the herbs on the tender body organs could have caused unwanted effects on the brain, liver and kidneys.

The common neonatal problems identified in babies in the first week post delivery were **dirty** and septic umbilical stumps.

Sources of support in baby care

Family members are a source of support and help postnatally. They help with baby care and promote breast feeding and allow a new mother time to rest. Although an elderly experienced member of the family is a valuable source of support for the new mother, sometimes there appears to be areas of conflict with the young mothers on principles of baby care, an aspect that confirms the need for professional advice and support postnatally. In contrast to suggestions on use of minimally trained health workers in the screening of post natal risk and management of post natal problems as suggested by (Raphael-Leff, 2003), the results of the small survey among Shona women in Harare suggested that women needed informed support from a knowledgeable source that could give convincing scientific information and explanation about self-care and baby care and could also upgrade the skills and information of the other members of the family.

Beliefs and Tradition in the Postnatal Period

Cultural beliefs, values and practices determine the health seeking behaviours of women in the postnatal period. Newborn care is based on these cultural beliefs(Abuidhail& Fleming,2007). There are varied practices from community to community on care of the newborn. It is important for the health practitioner to be aware of these in order to understand the behaviour around the newborn and to encourage the positive behaviours while discouraging negative practices. It is important to understand people's cultures and beliefs and the rationale behind the use of such practices in order to be able to advise appropriately. It is important that a health visitor is familiar with local traditions and practices.

Women were not familiar with physiological jaundice and this unusual feature generally caused panic among the new parents. The ingestion of bitter herbs by the newborn is widely believed by the Shona women's culture to prevent colicky abdominal pains. Some elderly women are disturbed by the presence of visible dark veins on a newborn's abdomen. They believe this feature is an abnormality, which must be treated by introducing herbs into the baby's system. Chewing roots and tree bark and introducing the sap through a kiss may transmit oral infections, thrush and tuberculosis to the newborn. Some babies have been made to ingest very strong doses of these substances resulting in diarrhoea with blood or causing death. New mothers and the elderly women in attention of the new mother can be informed of the safe and harmless practice of winding the baby after feeding to prevent abdominal colicky.

It is the responsibility of the health visitor to advise and inform families that babies are rarely born ill and do not need any "treatment" when they are born. The availability of vaccines and the immunisation schedule should be made known to the new parents who should be reassured of prevention of the known childhood preventable diseases. Availability of information on causes of disease in the newborn before the mother leaves hospital could be useful in allaying anxieties and preventing use of these harmful practices. In addition, availability of a professional support system at home ensures that the information is re-enforced and harmful practices are identified and discouraged. Some of the practices may become a source of conflict between the elderly and the young parents. Conflict in the new mother may trigger severe puerperal psychosis and unnecessary distress in the mother.

Critical Incident

A health visitor came across an elderly woman with several portions of traditional herbs one for each part of the body in time to diffuse a crisis that was imminent with the young daughter-in -law. According to the elderly lady, the baby's umbilicus was to be smeared with some greasy stuff to dry it off. The body was to be smeared with some green stuff to make the baby gain weight. A bundle of roots was to be chewed by granny's stained teeth and the sap introduced to the baby through a "kiss of life!" This was to make the baby strong and prevent colicky abdominal pains "typical of baby boys." Lastly and most important, the baby's genitals were to be "treated".

The old lady insisted she would treat her grandchild because this is how she had always managed all her sons including the baby's father. The daughter-in-law was found clutching her baby tightly on her chest, and obviously preventing the treatment session.

Some cultural practices not only expose the baby to infections like tetanus neonatorum, but may also interfere with successful feeding and may cause profuse haemorrhage and anaemia and body rash in the newborn. It is the duty of health personnel to understand their clients culture and advise on safe care practices.

The wide use of traditional practices for mother and child care could be an indication of an information void among the communities which health personnel must view as an unmet need for information. Health personnel must inform and equip their clients with safe health care skills. The impact of health information must constantly be assessed and approaches to imparting health information must be constantly revised in search of effective methods.

Critical Incident

Mrs. Hove delivered a bounty baby girl. She was discharged home and immediately her mother in law suggested Mrs. Hove should stay over with her until she picked up strength. When the midwife arrived to visit, Mrs.Hove's new born baby had been given a dose of tree bark sap. The baby was as flaccid as a rag doll with blood stained froth from the mouth and some of the "treatment" was coming out rectally. There were two jars of the subsequent doses concealed under the bed. The elderly lady disappeared when she was alerted of the midwife's arrival. Although this baby was rushed to hospital immediately, unfortunately she could not be saved.

Women's brief contact with health personnel when they visit the health institutions to have babies may not provide them with all the answers to the many postnatal questions and problems they have. A realistic assessment of the state of physical and mental health, economic and social status of a newly delivered mother is best done within her home environment so that the relevant suitable and appropriate assistance can be offered to her. Postnatal mothers are laden with hidden problems and anxieties which can only be known and assessed on a post natal home visit.

The common traditional practices among the newborn are out of fear of loosing the baby, especially where the family has lost a baby before. Anxiety to promote good digestion, raise a healthy heir, fear of witchcraft and jealousies from neighbours and wicked relatives are some reasons behind the practices. The health visitor must always show keenness to learn the meaning of cultural practices and be ready to provide scientific research based information to allay the mother's anxieties.

Baby Feeding and Growth Monitoring

Women living with elderly family members were reported to breast feed their babies. The care skills advocated by the elderly family members however often created conflicts between the young mothers and the elderly women as some of the practices were potentially dangerous. All women were encouraged to give their babies water to drink in between feeds, and some gave babies thin porridge to supplement inadequate breast milk (Murira,2006). Dehydration which was common among babies whose mothers lived on their own with the spouse was caused by reduced frequency to feed the baby and lack of skills to apply the baby to the breast.

Feeding babies with small amounts of water, honey and grounded filtered sugar, butter and minty water was also reported among some South Asian communities (Ingram, 2003; Fatmi et al.,2005). Such practices were believed to soften the meconeum and encourage the infant's bowels to move.

Ways of monitoring growth of the newborn, such as tying a string with a button around the baby's wrist, neck and waist have been observed among the Shona babies in Zimbabwe. Although these practices are harmless, care must be taken that the string does not become too tight around the arm and neck. The disadvantage of tying things around the body is that these strings absorb water during bath time and may cause chaffing and bruising around the neck, waist and wrists. Women should be informed of effective methods of growth monitoring such as attending regular baby weighing at the clinics and ensuring that the baby is well fed. A growth monitoring diary can be provided and mothers can participate in recording events in their babies' growth.

Warding off Evil Spirits

Some practices are thought to keep diseases and evil spirits away from the newborn. Thick necklace-like cloth strings with herbal powders or animal bone tied around the neck and waist may be unsightly as they collect sweat, saliva and dirt and may be a cause for chaffing around the neck and waist. Wet cloth necklaces may emit an unpleasant odour and may bruise the baby's neck. Health personnel should discourage these practices with care not to offend the mothers. Information on the immunisation against childhood diseases should be made available instead.

Steaming a baby under cover of a heavy blanket in dry herbal smoke or boiling herbal water to keep evil spirits away may choke the baby causing anoxia. Mothers should be equipped with information on safer baby care methods and especially to consult with health personnel when babies fall ill.

Eye Treatment

Women have been observed to spray the mother's milk into a discharging or indurated baby's eye. This practice is quite safe as the mother's milk is clean. This actually clears the eyes of dust or fluff.

Mothers should however be discouraged to use herbs and crushed leaves to clear discharge from the baby's eyes or to make the baby open his eyes. Introduction of herbs into the eyes may cause damage of varying degrees to the eyes resulting in poor eyesight or blindness. Mothers should be encouraged to seek health services where a baby's eyes has a discharge or looks sore. A pus swab should be taken and the baby commenced on antibiotics.

Umbilical "Care"

Elderly women have been observed to use herbs, sand, animal dung, and chicken droppings to seal to the umbilical stump. Elderly women use this practice out of fear of open wounds and out of anxiety to prevent bleeding and encourage quick drying of the wound. The mentioned substances have been strongly associated with tetanus neonatorum. Murira(2006) observed that the common neonatal problems identified among the Shona women were **dirty and septic umbilical stumps** with the use of "**herbal treatments**" on babies umbilical stumps. South Asian women were reported to use a mixture of ground lead to dry off the umbilicus (Abuildhail & Fleming,2007). It should be understood that clients engage in these practices because that is what they have always done and that they do not know of any alternatives. Clean and harmless methods of caring for the umbilical stump should be made known to the client and the relatives. It should be stressed to the client that cleaning the umbilical stump with alcohol or methylated spirits or boiled water and ensuring that it is mopped dry with each nappy change and each bath should be continued even after the stump has fallen off and is sealed.

Murira (2006) observed that elderly Shona women insisted on burying the dried umbilical stump as this was believed to preserve the new mother's fertility and bring luck to the newborn baby. Women must be given scientific information and explanation about unnecessary practices and beliefs and saved from engaging in unnecessary rituals.

Beauty and Tribal marks

Some tribes use 'decorative cuts' on the baby's face with razor blades and knives, in the hope of beautifying the baby or as a tribal identity. Decorative and tribal facial marks are common among some Nigerian, and Malawian tribes. South Asian women are reported to apply a ground lead to an infant's eyelids to make eyes beautiful (Fatmi et al.,2005). Health personnel should be on the alert and discourage such practices that may cause unnecessary pain on a helpless infant. Some of these invasive practices cause haemorrhage and infections such as tetanus and septicaemia. When the incisions heal, they may form ugly keloids and scar tissue that may cause health problems in later life. Some of these marks are so extensive that they leave ugly scars on the baby's face that amount to child abuse. Mothers and community elders must be informed of the pain inflicted on the small defenceless baby during these rituals and the danger of exposing the baby to haemorrhage, infection and possible loss of life.

Suppressing Sexual Hyperactivity

Spraying the genitals with the mother's milk is believed to subdue excessive desire for sexual activity in later life. This is a harmless practice believed to prevent promiscuity. Female infibulations however, at any age in life, is a dangerous, cruel and useless practice which should be strongly deplored and discouraged. This is harmful and senseless child abuse which must be reported to human rights authorities and police. Genital infibulations exposes the baby to haemorrhage, infection, contractures and the problems in reproduction later in life. Parents must be informed of these dangers and made to understand that sexual desire is normal and controlled by hormones not parts of the body.

Retracting the foreskin of the baby's penis every bath time is practised in some community. This practice may in fact cause cracks in the epithelial tissue of the foreskin resulting in phimosis and paraphimosis. Parents who advocate routine circumcision for baby boys can be advised that this procedure can be performed safely under sterile conditions by surgeons in hospitals and clinics. Some hospitals can perform this procedure within three days post delivery and before the baby leaves hospital for home.

External Rubs

External herbs or sap rubbed or massaged onto the baby's skin to encourage growth may be harmless to some babies but may cause irritating skin rash to others. A thick paste of herbs left in place over the anterior fontanel is believed to prevent illness in some cultures. While this maybe harmless to a certain extent, it may prevent the free breathing of pores of the scalp. Parents should be informed of childhood preventable diseases and encouraged to take their infants for immunizations to prevent childhood diseases.

Speeding up Development

Some cultures make razor incisions on the baby's joints and these are packed with various powders from animal and plants believed to encourage quick development of the infant from one milestone to the other. Postnatal health education should discourage practices that break the newborn's skin exposing the infant to several blood and skin infections. It is imperative that health personnel provide information on factors that promote growth and development in the baby such as prevention of infection, good feeding routines, and gradual introduction of baby foods. Parents should be advised on observing expected growth milestones and early identification of developmental abnormalities.

Cultural beliefs, values and practices have a great influence on the care of infants in many cultures. The midwife/health visitor must respect the women's culture and familiarise herself with prevalent practices on infants in order to identify the practices that may have a negative impact on the development of the newborn infant. Knowledge of potentially dangerous practices enables the health visitor to give appropriate health information and advice and to persuade the parents to desist from such practices.

The need for research

Health professionals must continuously engage in research in newborn care and continuously seek new information and approaches to various aspects of care in order to improve the quality of mother and child care. Constant reviews and reflections on mother and child care and invitation of women to actively participate in recommended methods of self-care and baby care should be encouraged to raise the quality of women's health and that of the newborn infants.

References

1. Abuildhail,J.,Fleming,V. Beliefs and practices of postpartum infant care:review of different cultures. British Journal of Midwifery,2007,15(7) 418-421

2. Murira,N. Pregnancy, Labour, Self-Care and Baby Care. Publish America, 2006. Maryland USA.

3. Thomson, A. Learning from the community about barriers to health care. *Obstetrics and Gynaecology,* 1997; 87 (1):140-141.

4. WHO Prevention and Care of illness- neonates and infants. WHO(2004) Geneva

5. Fatmi,Z.,Gulzar,A.Z., Kazi,A. Maternal and Newborn Care: practices and beliefs of traditional birth attendants in Sindhi,Pakistan. Eastern Mediterranean Journal, 2005,11(1/2): 226-234

6. Ingram,,J., Johnson,D.,Hamid,NSouth Asian grandmothers'influence on breastfeeding in Bristol. Midwifery,2003,19:318-327

7. Murira, N., Lützen, K., Lindmark, G. and Christensson K. (2003). Communication patterns between health personnel and their clients in an antenatal clinic in Zimbabwe. *Journal of Women's Health.* 24(2), pp. 83-92.

8. Murira, N. (2006). *Pregnancy, Labour, Self-Care and Baby Care.* Maryland, USA: Publish America.

9. Murira,N.Communicating sexual and reproductive health messages. In search of a model to increase risk perception among primiparous women. PhD Thesis.2010 Birmingham City University.

10. Raphael-Leff (2003)Psycological Process of Chid-bearing. London: Chapman Hall

CHAPTER 11

WHAT DO WOMEN WANT?

Unless health personnel engage women in wide discussions and consultation about their health needs, and understand the cultural beliefs, superstition, fears and practices, they cannot address the causes of maternal and neonatal morbidity and mortality adequately. Health personnel may not plan effective interventions without this knowledge and health advice may not be appreciated.

The feminine culture worldwide however emphasizes self- preparation to be attractive, desirable and useful to men even outside the child birth milieu. This cultural rule is enforced without necessarily putting it into words (Bryar, 1995). One psychologist expressed the societal expectations of the woman as follows:

> *"It is natural and inevitable for young women to be anxious and sometimes frightened of adulthood because the culturally defined roles for women place opposing and incompatible demands on young women. Young women are expected to meet their traditional role, to be attractive, dependent, and affectionate and family oriented while being expected to meet expectations of independence and success in the public sphere"* (Lee, 1998).

Shaping up

Women desire to look good throughout pregnancy and immediately post delivery. Research has revealed that at each stage of the woman's progression or development along the child bearing phase, there are specific exercises a woman has to be aware of that focus on the bodily changes taking place during the specific times and the body's needs (Balaskas, 1989; Robertson, 1997). Exercise requirements in the child bearing phase can therefore be arranged to suit women in the preconception period, first trimester, second trimester, third or final trimester and the post natal period.

Contrary to the cultural beliefs, physical exercises in pregnancy do not adversely affect pregnancy but promotes good circulation and improves lung ventilation which is good for the pregnant woman (Gross & Pattison, 2007). Exercises prevent stasis of venous blood that causes varicose veins. Good flow of maternal blood promotes good placental blood circulation.

Exercises improve the tone of muscles preventing sagging and flabby muscles. Being shapely is part of womanhood and femininity and making oneself attractive and desirable to the partner is culture based (Lee, 1998). Active young adults are believed to have healthy pregnancies and easy childbirth.

'Culture is obsessed with appearance. In some cultures, loss of weight post delivery is equated to self control. Bodily perfection is equated to moral perfection. Physical beauty is a result of hard work, ambition and self control. The overweight are what they are because they are lazy to do something about their weight and are self indulgent' (Lee, 1998).

Exercises throughout the child bearing phase are designed to suit the physiological changes in pregnancy and the recuperation post delivery (Balaskas, 1989). Exercises in pregnancy are cumulative and carried over from one trimester to the next. It is important that midwives and health visitors work hand in hand with physiotherapists to engage women in phase specific exercises.

Post delivery, women need to engage in exercises to return to shape and to shed off the massive weight gained during pregnancy. Women openly express their desire to be shapely post delivery and indicate some of the parts of their bodies they desire to reduce in size. In some cultures women tie their abdomens tightly with pieces of cloth to control the abdominal flab in the hope of quickly regaining the pre-pregnancy shape. Elderly women too encourage tying the abdominal muscles to prevent the flab that occurs post delivery. Shona women's culture is concerned that the empty abdomen post delivery may fill up with wind, hence the need to tie a cloth around the waist. Young women comply with this practice out of fear of collection of large amounts of wind in the abdomen and also because of anxiety to regain the pre-pregnancy shape as quickly as possible post delivery. The tight belt is kept in place for at least 6-8 weeks post delivery.

Tying the abdominal muscles is probably meant to serve the same purpose a modern girdle or corset serves; the difference is that the corset stretches and allows for muscle movement. The corset embraces and supports all abdominal muscles, hip and thighs whereas the tight piece of cloth is around the waist like a belt. Women have indicated that they are instructed by elderly women to tie the abdomen.

'I was told to tie this tight band around my abdomen until my abdomen is back to normal.'

.'I was told to tie the abdomen tightly preferably with the baby's nappy to expel wind which collects in the abdomen to occupy the space previously occupied by the baby.

"I have nothing to wear because all my clothes do not fit so I have no choice but to use this tight belt."(Murira,2010)

The practice of tying the abdomen of a newly delivered woman with a tight cloth is combined with taking a beverage made from crushed herbs from the bark of specific trees known for their bitterness which is thought to contract the abdominal muscles. It is not easy to figure out how a beverage contracts specific muscles in the body; the women do not know either but believe the magical powers of the beverage. Young first time mothers are victims of cultural practices as they are instructed to follow orders from their mentors. Water is continuously added to the crushed bark until the once bitter beverage becomes tasteless or until the bark becomes mouldy and smelly. These practices can be interpreted as a desperate expression of trying to regain shape post delivery. The desperate practices to reshape the body post delivery justify the need for creating awareness in women on the process of involution. Post natal exercises should ideally be commenced immediately after delivery to prevent lung complications and thrombo-embolic diseases and to tone up muscles (Robetson,1997; Hillsdon et al, 2005;Murira,2006).

The Importance of Exercise

Health personnel have a duty to communicate health promoting information to encourage speedy recovery of women from effects of pregnancy. The role of exercise in promoting recuperation post delivery and promoting good health everyday cannot be overemphasized.

Exercise is important for improvement of general physical fitness. As one exercises one's body, the stored fats and carbohydrates burn up and are used as energy. One loses excess water and wastes from the body through sweat. Exercises strengthen and tone muscles and encourage improved shape, stable gait and good posture.

Exercise in general is important for movement of body joints, improves muscle and joint movement and prevents bad posture, stiff joints and general aches and pains. Exercise is important in maintaining good body balance especially post pregnancy where one needs to gradually loose body weight. Activity improves blood flow, makes the heart to beat harder and faster pumping blood to all parts of the body. Through exercises, sagging smooth muscles are tightened, fluid sitting in wrong places in the body is moved and oedema in parts of the body like the limbs and waist reduces.

The increase in the breathing rate during exercises draws in more air to the lungs, which expand to the maximum. The fresh air is passed onto the blood as the blood gives off carbon dioxide from muscle activity. The fresh blood prevents muscle cramps and promotes tissue repair and healing. Regular exercise post delivery heals the body restores the body to the pre-pregnancy state and keeps the body healthy.

Post delivery, women must be encouraged to gradually take exercises to a higher level to tone up muscles weakened by the effect of pregnancy hormones. The abdominal muscles stretched in pregnancy regain their tone with regular exercise. The extra weight gained due to cravings in pregnancy is burnt up through regular exercises.

Post delivery, after engaging in more demanding exercises, one sleeps well, and wakes up refreshed and with renewed energy.

Exercise improves appetite post delivery as one burns up stored energy, the body demands for food intake and one's appetite improves. A woman needs good nutrition that contains protein for repair of tissues worn out or bruised during pregnancy and labour. One needs a diet rich in vitamins, minerals such as iron, calcium to improve lowered levels of blood components during pregnancy and labour and for healthy breast feeding.

When is the best time to exercise?

Exercises are more effective if done first thing in the morning. Exercise done first thing in the morning is refreshing as the lungs fill with fresh cool air before the air is polluted by suit and smog from domestic, industrial and vehicle fumes. Women must be advised to exercise for a short period until they feel stronger and one's body adjusts to the workout. Gradually one can increase the time spent exercising and vary the types of exercises. Women who are known to suffer from heart disease should seek the doctor's advice before engaging in a vigorous exercise routine. If however a woman feels very tired, she must be investigated to exclude anaemia and other underlying conditions.

Women must be advised to exercise before a meal. The heart cannot cope with digesting a heavy meal as well as coping with exercise! It is best to start with simple exercises and gradually increase the variety of the exercise until one feels strong enough to join local joggers in one's area or go to the local gym and to the 'Keep Fit' group exercises

Whether exercises are during pregnancy or post delivery, women can team up with their partner and enjoy the advantages of exercise. Women feel supported and encouraged if the partner teams up with them. Post delivery the weight gained in pregnancy becomes a burden. Gradual loss of weight that excludes starvation and stringent diets is advisable to enable the heart to cope with the reduced volume of body mass. Health personnel must advise women on sensible ways to reduce weight. Crush diets are unhealthy for the heart. Crush diets cause electrolyte imbalance and essential food elements in the body system leading to conditions like anaemia, eating disorders, and ulcers. A woman needs a good diet to recover from effects of pregnancy and labour and be able to take up new responsibilities as a mother and strength to breast feed and produce adequate milk for the baby.

A balanced diet low in fats and carbohydrates but rich in fruit and vegetables and protein is ideal to replace lost fluids and electrolytes, and for successful breastfeeding and repair of bruised tissues. Vitamins which are abundant in fruits and vegetables are essential for tissue repair, replenishing the haemoglobin and prevention of infection, while proteins are essential in the diet for repair of tissues.

Stretch Marks

Stretch marks post delivery disappears with the tightening of the abdominal muscles. Engaging in postnatal exercises soon after delivery helps to tone the muscles and rid the abdomen of the marked stretch marks.

Postnatal mothers can take up physical exercises as soon as the aches and pains of labour fade away. Deep breathing exercises ensure cardio-respiratory fitness and prevent pulmonary embolism and hypostatic pneumonia, while pelvic floor muscle exercises tone up the overstretched pelvic floor muscles (Hillsdom et al.,2005). Leg exercises are encouraged immediately post delivery to prevent stasis of blood in the lower legs and the resultant deep vein thrombosis due to prolonged bed rest post delivery.

Exercises can be held in a particular venue for post natal mothers to enable the mothers to interact with the midwife and get information on health problems. This arrangement may not be convenient for all women, some of whom may prefer to engage in a programme that suits their specific needs. Discussion with individual women will enable the midwife to assist each woman to adopt a programme that suites her needs.

Toning Abdominal Muscles

The abdominal muscles are attached to the back, and along the centre of the abdomen and the pelvis in front. During pregnancy the abdominal muscles stretch forward to accommodate the growing uterus. The muscles also pull on the back, changing the body structure and increasing the chances of a backache. After delivery abdominal muscles remain loose, bulky and flabby until the woman tones them.

Toning abdominal muscles post delivery can be done this way:

- The woman can start with simple deep breathing in and out. Deep breathing post delivery helps to expel blood from the womb.

- Deep breathing expands the lungs preventing lung complications especially **hypostatic pneumonia.**

- The woman can lie down flat on her back with legs together and stretched. She stretches her arms above her head. She breathes in pulling in her abdominal muscles as she further stretches her arms and legs as far as possible. Repeat five to ten times.

- The woman puts her hands on her side. She bends the left leg and puts the foot of the bent leg flat on the floor.

- Keeping her right leg straight, she lifts it up as high as possible towards her tummy and puts it down. Repeat ten times. Repeat these movements with the left leg while bending the right leg. This exercise tones the back, buttocks, thighs and pelvic floor muscles.

- Lying flat on the floor, the woman bends one knee and pulls it up over her abdomen as far as she can go. She repeats ten times with each leg. This exercise firms thighs, abdominal muscles and pelvic floor muscles.

- The woman sits up with legs stretched out and astride. She stretches her arms outwards. Tucks her tummy in as she stretches the right arm across to reach for her toes of the left foot ten times. She must do the same with the left arm touching the toes on the right foot.

- Ask the woman to go on fours with knees and arms apart. She breathes in pulling in her abdominal muscles stretching out her shoulders like an angry cat then breathes out repeatedly for five to ten times.
- The woman stands up with her feet astride. Swings her arms from side to side ten times to each side. This movement tightens the rings of muscles that look like flat tyres under the arms and upper abdomen.

Abdominal muscles may remain flabby for a long time after delivery. Many women anxious to regain their pre-pregnancy shape may resort to tying the abdomen with tight belts, napkins or any piece of material (Murira, 2010). Women should be persuaded to desist from this practice that interferes with good blood floor, instead they should be encouraged to engage in post natal exercises that tone the abdominal muscles.

The abdominal muscles are by far more exposed to overstretching in pregnancy than any other muscle in the body. They loose shape and tone and many women may find it most difficult to regain their pre-pregnancy abdominal tone. The **rectus abdominis** muscle, the **transverse abdominis**, the internal and external oblique are extensively stretched to accommodate the growing uterus. Exercises to this part of the body are meant to tone the muscles and contract them back to shape.

Breathing

This is an exercise that can be commenced immediately post delivery. Deep breathing assists the abdominal muscles to gain their tone. Deep breathing also contracts the uterus and pushes it down into the pelvis where it belongs. Breathing in and out can be done in any position a client can decide to be, lying down on a flat surface, legs straight and arms straight against the body. In that position, arms can be stretched up as legs are stretched downwards to give the rectus abdominis a good stretch and relaxation that improves the muscle tone.

Abdominal Tuck

Lying on a flat surface, with knees bent, the abdominal muscles are pulled in, the back is pushed firmly against the floor, as one takes in a deep breath, counts up to five, then breathes out.

Abdominal muscle contraction

From a lying position, knees bent, arms straight against the body, one brings the chin and chest slowly towards the abdomen, without the support of the elbows. Slowly one moves the trunk back to the flat position. Repeat 5-10 times. When the muscles are toned up, it is easy to bring the chest and knees together over the abdomen.

Leg and abdomen combined contraction

Lying flat, hands on the sides, one bends one leg at knee level and brings it over the abdomen as far as possible assisted by the arms, and to a straight position. Repeat five times and change to the other leg. With both legs bent, repeat movement. Build up the movements to a count up to ten. This exercise not only tones the abdomen, but the thigh muscles and the pelvic floor muscles as well.

Clients who have delivered by Caesarean Section may not participate in some of the exercises a woman who had a normal delivery may engage in. They may need to allow the Caesarean wound to heal before engaging in vigorous exercises. They may not engage in exercises that stress their abdominal muscles until at least six weeks after delivery when healing of the wound is presumed to be at an advanced stage. It is advisable to consult with the doctor or physiotherapist.

Pelvic Floor Muscle exercise

The pelvic floor consists of the *levator ani* muscles (the pubic portion and the iliac portion). The vaginal orifice and the rectum perforate these muscles. *The levator ani*, inferiorly meet with the *levator coccygeus* muscle and *the piriformis* muscle to form the perineal body. These muscles are subjected to extensive stretching during the perineal phase of labour and may be bruised and torn at the end of the second stage of labour.

The pelvic floor muscles fan out to form a hammock that holds the pelvic contents, the urinary bladder, the uterus and ovaries, the large bowel. It is important that these muscles return to shape and acquire a good tone to hold the pelvic contents in place.

Pelvic floor muscle exercise should be regarded as a lifetime exercise to prevent such complications as prolapse of female pelvic organs and stress incontinence in later life.

Loss of tone of pelvic floor muscles may be noticed by failure to hold urine which may dribble when laughing or coughing. Toning pelvic floor muscles is an exercise that can be done anywhere anytime and does not need preparation. It does not disturb a woman's work or any of her routines.

Pelvic floor muscle exercises can be done at any time in any position. Women should therefore find it easy to continue toning this very important group of muscles to prevent bladder, uterine or rectal prolapse and stress incontinence in later years.

- A woman pretends that her bladder is full and that she has an urge to empty it but you cannot find a toilet. She must pinch her muscles tight down below without squeezing her buttocks or moving her legs together then pull the muscles inwards for a count of three and relaxes the muscles.

- This exercise can be repeated up to a count of ten whenever one wishes. Women must continue this exercise throughout pregnancy. This exercise can be done when having sex; it enhances the partner's and the woman's sexual enjoyment!

- Post delivery; pelvic floor exercise must be taken to another level.

- A woman must pretend that a soggy tampon is about to drop or that she has a runny tummy but the toilet is a distance away. She must pull the muscles in as if to keep the tampon in and to prevent the bowel from opening.

- A woman must start exercising soon after delivery to tone the loose pelvic floor muscles.

- After the muscle relaxation caused by the pregnancy hormones, the stretch caused by the weight of the baby in late pregnancy and the stretch during delivery, the pelvic floor muscles need serious attention and toning up.

- The movements of the pelvic floor muscles must be continued as before but this time around the woman is encouraged to pull the muscles in and hold for a count up to five. She must exercise more frequently and also assess how good her efforts are.

Assessing the tone of the pelvic floor muscles:

- Immediately after delivery, the pelvic floor muscles are very loose. As the woman takes a bath she must try this exercise and will notice that the birth canal is wide open. An index finger stuck in the birth canal while bathing may not be gripped by contracting pelvic floor muscles. As one continues the exercise one should gradually feel the birth canal muscles grip the index finger as one exercises. That is the first stage of toning up the muscles.

- Toning up of the muscles must continue until the muscles can grip the small finger! This is the second stage of pelvic floor muscle toning.
- The final stage is stopping the urine flow as one is half way emptying the bladder. One should be able to hold urine for a while then continue to empty the remaining amount. When one reaches this stage, one must continue to exercise throughout her lifetime to maintain this pelvic floor muscle tone.

What happens if pelvic floor muscles remain loose?

- Loose pelvic floor muscles can cause urine leaks and dribbles meaning that a woman will always need a pad to receive the dribble.
- The woman is likely to always smell of urine, which makes her very uncomfortable and causes loss of confidence.
- Pelvic organs can slip out through the loose muscles as one coughs, sneezes, lifts heavy objects or pushes a bowel motion. This is called   prolapse of pelvic organs.
- **A woman can have a uterine prolapse, a rectal prolapse or a bladder prolapse.**
- A pelvic organ prolapse is a serious condition that is uncomfortable and embarrassing to live with. One is prone to infection which may cause a nasty smell.
- Organ prolapse may be corrected by intensive pelvic floor muscle exercises. A rubber ring pushed up the vaginal wall can be used in uterine prolapse but the problem can be corrected permanently through surgery.

Thigh Trimming

In pregnancy, excess carbohydrates and fats are deposited in fat depots under the skin in such areas as the thighs and buttocks. The skin over these areas becomes dimpled and puckered to look like an orange peel due to the fat and water, cellulite, trapped underneath. In order to fight against cellulite, a combination of a good diet and exercises is required. It is advisable to reduce on the intake of fats and carbohydrates, salt, sugar, alcohol and increase the intake of protein, water, fruit and vegetables. Post delivery exercises of thigh muscles reduces the size of thighs, firm the thighs so that they lose the flabbiness caused by pregnancy hormones.

Thigh firming exercises include:

- **Standing up astride left hand on the hip,** right hand stretched out then stretching out the left leg in kicking movements as high as possible to reach out on the fingers of the stretched hand ten times then change to the right leg.

This exercise tones the back, the abdominal muscles, and pelvic floor muscles and improves circulation in legs reducing swelling in legs.

- Bend the left knee to meet the bent right elbow in kicking movements ten times then do the same with the right leg.
- Stand up behind a chair and rest arms on the back of the chair with legs as wide apart as possible. Bend both knees slowly and slowly move the trunk downwards keeping the back straight. Hold the body in that position and feel the thigh muscles tighten up. Slowly pull the body up and repeat movements up to five times.
- When one feels strong and able to withstand the programmed rhythmic exercises one can join the local 'Keep Fit Group'.
- Remember to keep fit one must eat a balanced diet. Weight gain is gradual so is weight loss.

One can engage in simple exercises like

- **Brisk walking** initially for twenty minutes and gradually increased as one gets used to the exercise is not only effective but enjoyable.
- If one has access to stairs, **stepping up and down two steps** until one feels an ache in the thighs is also good exercise.
- **Lying flat on the floor,** one leg is lifted a few centimeters from the floor and one slowly draws circles in the air fife times before shifting to the opposite leg.
- **Still lying flat on the floor,** one lifts one leg up to a vertical position and down to the floor in quick succession for a count of up to fife and shifts to the other leg. One should be able to build up on the counts with time up to a count of ten before exercising the other leg.
- **Scissors movements.** With both legs lifted a few centimeters from the floor, one moves the legs up and down in opposite directions like a pair of scissors. This exercise also tones up the abdominal muscles and the perineal muscles.
- **Cycling.** From the above position one moves the legs as if cycling for a count up to ten.

- **Lying on the side and resting on one elbow,** lift the top most leg up and down until the thigh aches then change sides.

- **Standing astride,** stretch one hand out and aim to kick it with the opposite leg. Repeat movement ten times before changing to the other leg.

- **Standing upright,** bending one arm, lift the opposite knee to touch the bent elbow alternating the legs all the time. Repeat ten times.

- **Jogging.** In order to do this exercise, a check up of blood pressure and heart condition is necessary. One can jog on the spot or for a distance starting with fife minutes and building up as the body gets used to the exercise.

Dancing

One enjoyable way to loose weight and stay slim is to engage in regular dancing. The different strides, stretches and postures adopted in dancing help to reduce weight while one is having fun. It is through a planned system of continuous contact between health personnel and women that women can be supported, advised and informed about how they can look after themselves post delivery.

References

1. Balaskas, J. (1989). *Active Birth*. London: Unwin Paperbacks.
2. Bryar, R.M. (1995). *Theory for Midwifery Practice*. London: Macmillan Publishing.
3. Gross, H. and Pattison, H. (2007). *Sanctioning Pregnancy. A Psychological Perspective on the Paradoxes and Culture of Research*. London: Routledge
4. Hillsdon, M., Foster, C. and Thorogood, M. (2005). Interventions for promoting physical activity. *Cochrane Database of Systematic Reviews*. (1), CD003180.
5. Lee, C. (1998). *Women's Health: Psychological and Social Perspectives*. California: Sage Publications
6. Murira,N.Communicating sexual and reproductive health messages: In search of a model to increase risk perception among primiparous women. PhD Thesis (2010) Birmingham City University
7. Murira, N. (2006). *Pregnancy, Labour, Self-Care and Baby Care*. Maryland, USA: Publish America.
8. Robertson,(1997)

Chapter 12

HEALTH PROMOTION

Adults need information to solve their immediate problems. Women need information that responds to their current pressing needs so that they can solve their health problems (Brookfield, 1986). Information given as the women approach each phase along the child-bearing process helps women to understand the phase better and cope with the demands of the specific phase confidently. Women need information that they can use in the post partum period for their self care and baby care. Information needs are varied from one woman to another. Young first time mothers need support in self- care and baby care skills. Some information needs women may need post delivery are breast care, wound care, family planning, weight loss and baby care. It is therefore imperative that health personnel communicate effectively with each woman to identify each woman's personal information needs.

Primiparous women in developed countries are reported to be satisfied with health information they receive on leaving health institutions (Hunter, 2008). This is in contrast to most African women who have little or no information on discharge from health institutions. The contrast in information available to women in developed and developing countries suggests that with commitment among health personnel, it is possible for health personnel to provide information to the satisfaction of one's clientele. Communication is an attitude that can be learnt, developed and evaluated with commitment (ten Carte,2000).

Contraception Post Delivery

Whereas in the pre-pregnancy period, there seems to be an irrational rush by young women to fall pregnant, postnatally, women are keen to use contraception and enquire about it expressing the desire to use long term family planning methods (Murira,2010). This behavior suggests that fertility is a universal human concern and the ability of women in most cultures to nurture a pregnancy and have a successful delivery is considered the essence of being a complete woman (Helman, 2001). Reports from various societies indicate that proof of fertility and successful pregnancy makes women desire to control their fertility post delivery (Dow & Werner, 1981;Ekabua et al.,2004; Aisen et al.,2004;Hunter,2008).

Suggestions have been made that at such times when women are ready to accept contraception, information on effective methods of family planning should be made available to women so to enable them to make informed choice on the contraception methods (Sanogo et al., 2003). Postnatally women are more receptive to family planning information as the statements below suggest.

> 'I want a reliable long acting family planning method"
>
> 'I do not wish to fall pregnant for a long time to come so I want a reliable method'
>
> 'I want to go back to school so I want to use a good family planning method.'
>
> 'I need to look after my baby well without distractions before adding another sibling.
>
> I don't want to   fall pregnant soon and experience the pain of labour again so soon.'(Murira,2010)

Postnatal family planning service is a vital component of reproductive health service that ensures that new mothers have information to make an informed choice on available and suitable family planning methods to postpone another pregnancy. A reliable method of family planning is desirable especially after a pregnancy to allow the woman a reasonable time to recover from the effects of the previous pregnancy and the stress of labour. It is also important that mothers postpone pregnancy until the new baby is fairly independent.

Midwives and health visitors should assess women's current knowledge of family planning to add new information on the woman's existing knowledge. Health personnel should discuss and explain fully to the women the family planning methods available and how these work to enable women to make informed choices of contraceptive methods they may wish to use.

 It is reported that women in some parts of Africa, face community disapproval and husband control on issues related to fertility and this prevents them from exercising their family planning choices (Barnett et al.,1999). Reports from some parts of Africa indicate that male supremacy controls women's reproductive lives and yet African men are generally poorly informed on issues related to fertility and pregnancy (Aina et al, 2002; Mesfin, 2002; Kabir et al,2003). Through domiciliary visits and community education, negative attitudes towards family planning can change allowing women an opportunity to exercise their family planning choices.

Post delivery, it is important that health personnel assess young women's family planning knowledge, attitudes and practices in family planning to enable advising them appropriately. More detailed research needs to be done to monitor the changes in knowledge, attitudes and practices in family planning use in young teenage mothers. The availability of family planning methods may not be sufficient to encourage use of family planning methods by young men and women. Health visitors should provide information about how the methods work and can be used, and information that addresses negative community attitudes and misconceptions about family planning use.

Sexual Relationships Post delivery

In some cultures women may have hesitancy to resume sexual intercourse until after six weeks or longer. In such cultures, the women's culture seems to stipulate time for resumption of sexual activities. The stipulated time to refrain from sexual activity is not based on evidence but women 's culture seems to have an emphasis on the young woman showing complete recovery and gaining strength to look after themselves and the baby before being allowed to live with their spouses. This practice lengthens the period of spousal separation. The rationale behind this practice seems to lie in the belief that a frail woman is not useful to the man and family and that post delivery a woman needs rest and a good diet to enable healing in preparation for the responsibility ahead. Men in such cultures accept that they can only live with the woman when she is ready for her womanly duties, when she is healed and strong and ready to start the cycle of reproduction once more. Some common attitudes about resumption of sex post delivery are revealed through these statements from primiparous women :

> ' I have been told by my grandmother that I cannot have sexual relations before two months elapse; it will affect my baby.'
>
> "I can't think of sexual intercourse now, I am still very sore. Besides, my grandmother says I have to wait for about three months before living with my partner again."
>
> 'My grandmother told me to wait till I am strong.'(Murira, 2010).

The spousal separation in the Shona culture seems to serve three purposes, namely; that it allows the woman time to heal; it enables recuperation and it delays another pregnancy too soon. The postnatal spousal separation among the Shona couples is a continuation of separation from twenty-eight weeks of gestation when abstention from sexual activity is meant to prevent 'injury' to the unborn baby until the culture stipulates the ideal time for sexual activity post delivery. Fear inducing messages of adverse consequences if one breaches the elderly women's advice compels the young women to comply with the advice.

The prolonged spousal separation practised post delivery by some communities however exposes couples to the already high prevalence of sexually transmitted diseases including HIV /AIDS. Extra marital sexual activities are reported in some studies to be rife during spousal sexual abstinence in the postnatal period (Blanc & Sage, 2000) when women abstain from sexual activity but their husbands are not sanctioned by any cultural law or belief to abstain from sexual activity. Through the abstention practices women's culture enforces cultural rules that disadvantage fellow women and expose women and their spouses to risk (Madebwe & Madebwe,2006). After the stipulated period of sexual abstinence and the couple is allowed to live together, the spouse is expected to practise 'safe sex' in the form of coitus interruptus to prevent early pregnancy.

Preventing Unplanned Pregnancy

Early return to pre-pregnant hormonal activity and possible ovulation resulting in unplanned pregnancies surprises many young mothers. Health personnel are encouraged to discuss Family planning methods in the presence of the spouses where possible so that both partners get an opportunity to participate in the discussion and ask questions to enable them to make an informed decision. Many women believe they may not fall pregnant as long as they breast feed. Information on the menstrual cycle, and how ovulation easily occurs as levels of oxytocin decline post delivery should be explained in a simple but convincing way to the mother. Health personnel should advise couples to embark on a reliable family planning method just before the lochia dries out completely and before the couple indulges in active sexual activity.

Taboos

It is important that health personnel are familiar with their clients' culture so that they can provide culture sensitive advice. Murira,(2010) observed that women not all foods were considered good for the postnatal mother. Newly delivered women were subjected to nutritional taboos and compelled to observe food taboos some of which were the only readily available source of protein, iron, minerals, vitamins and roughage at a time when the women needed these foods for their personal recovery and for successful breastfeeding.

Some cultures advised the young newly delivered women should eat well but foods had to be approved by the elderly women. Post delivery, in some cultures, women are advised to eat for two as food eaten by the mother is believed to 'flow' to her baby through the milk. Murira,(2010) observed that postnatal women were encouraged to eat a lot of the carbohydrate rich staple foods, home made high protein beverages made of millet and salted nuts to keep the milk flowing. Women were however not allowed to eat eggs and beans as eggs were believed to make the baby fretful and the beans would delay baby's teething process. It is important that health visitors enquire on the dietary practices expected of women post delivery in order to provide evidence based advice that promotes speedy recovery and good health of the postnatal mother.

Fig.12.1 Concepts of Femininity in the post natal period(Murira,2010)

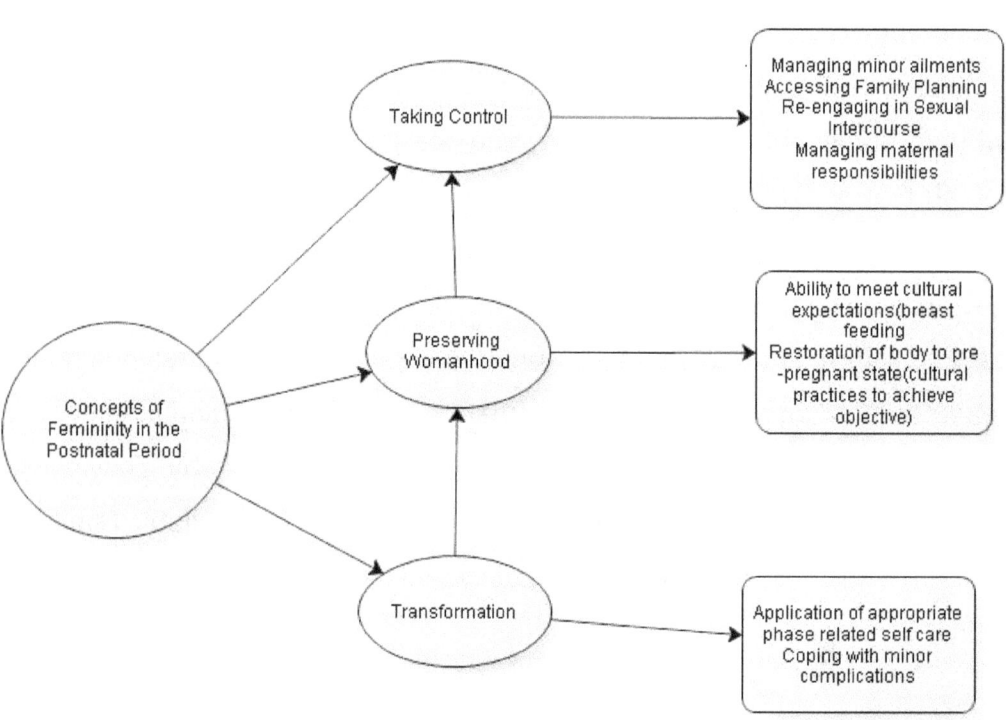

The postnatal period is a critical period for both mother and child. Health personnel must be at hand to provide effective health promotion information for self-care and care of the infant as well as to promote family good health in general. Health personnel must make efforts to reduce post natal morbidity through a planned and structured maternal and infant health monitoring system which enables prevention of chronic ill health in women.

Risk Perception in the Post Partum Period

Culture helps one to understand risk in a particular cultural context and this is a communal notion of risk and not an individualistic view. Culture determines which risks are high risks worth worrying about (Lupton, 1999). In the postnatal period, culture plays a significant role in the management of the puerperium. Women who fail to access professional advice as an alternative to cultural teaching rely fully on their tradition and culture resulting in women failing to identify risks to their health. In the absence of evidence based information, clients' awareness of risk can only be understood from a socio-cultural point of view which is unlikely to bear similar meanings of the severity of risk and is unlikely to pay the risk the urgency it deserves. The clients are unlikely to adopt appropriate health behaviours that promote good health, they may not be aware of risk are unlikely to apply effective self-care skills.

Without professional advice, women may practise what comes naturally to them, what they know, what is easy and affordable to them and what they can get support in. Where women have no perception of risk, they may not take precautions to prevent risks because they do not perceive the risks. There may be no attempts to seek health care services. It is possible that the elderly women have no knowledge about reproductive health complications and are unaware of the implications of the complications to women's health.

Where there is a general lack of basic knowledge of what constitutes 'risk' in both the young women and their mentors, the absence of a back up health service in the form of a domiciliary postnatal service, and the non-existence of complementary leaflets and books to empower women with information, women are exposed to high reproductive risk that exposes them to morbidity and mortality in the postnatal period.

Development of cultural awareness among health personnel cannot be overemphasized as it enables free interact with women and recognition of the women's values, beliefs and practices. Cultural awareness requires that health personnel engage in frequent friendly interaction with women and learn from the women's culture. It may be worthwhile for health personnel to consider engaging the women's mentors in a discussion and process of information exchange as a way of influencing the beliefs, values and practices of women.

Where health personnel-client communication is poor, women leave health services unaware of risks they are exposed to at each stage of the child bearing process from pregnancy, labour and the post natal period. Women will not be prepared for the events that follow the delivery of their babies. Primiparous women are generally young and inexperienced and may not have knowledge of the physiology of the puerperium and involution. In their communities, young women are made to believe that all should be well after delivery of the baby. The young women are therefore alarmed by post delivery negative events such as post partum haemorrhage and other complications.

However, the women's culture is 'organized' and has behavioural objectives clearly spelt out by the cultural ethos (Webb, 1986). Women go back to their cultural practices and pursue their expected child-bearing cultural practices oblivious of the impact the behaviour has on their health and the health of their newly born babies. In their home environments, the young teenage primiparous women depend on mature 'uninformed' women of the community for care and support, information needs, and reassurance. This is an aspect that the health sector in many African countries has to address as a matter of urgency in order to reduce maternal morbidity and mortality.

Young inexperienced women can become easy targets of ineffective and potentially dangerous cultural perinatal practices such as use of herbs inserted in the birth canal and invasive lactation stimulants which cause breast engorgement and breast abscesses. Women may develop complications and fail to understand them and take appropriate action to manage these complications. Young women cannot challenge potentially dangerous cultural practices such as extended separation from their spouses, a likely source of sexually transmitted diseases including HIV/AIDS because they are not informed of the impact of such practices.

In the absence of professional support, women apply the practices they believe can restore womanhood according to their feminine cultural beliefs and practices (Kavanagh and Kennedy, 1992; Helman, 2001). Health personnel should embrace the women's culture as one strategy that could effectively assist women to increase risk perception as research confirms that understanding clients' cultures forms the central linchpin to understanding the health behaviours of women in the child-bearing phase (Leineinger, 2005).

Research has revealed that cultural practices are rife in clients' homes away from health personnel and the young women have no choice but to comply with the rituals because there are no alternative forms of care available to them(Murira,2010). Health personnel may not be aware of this aspect of the women's culture, which has real potential to increase morbidity and mortality.

Figure 12.2 illustrates how teenage primiparous women without effective knowledge of the childbearing process and professional support during the post natal period can be exposed to post natal risk.

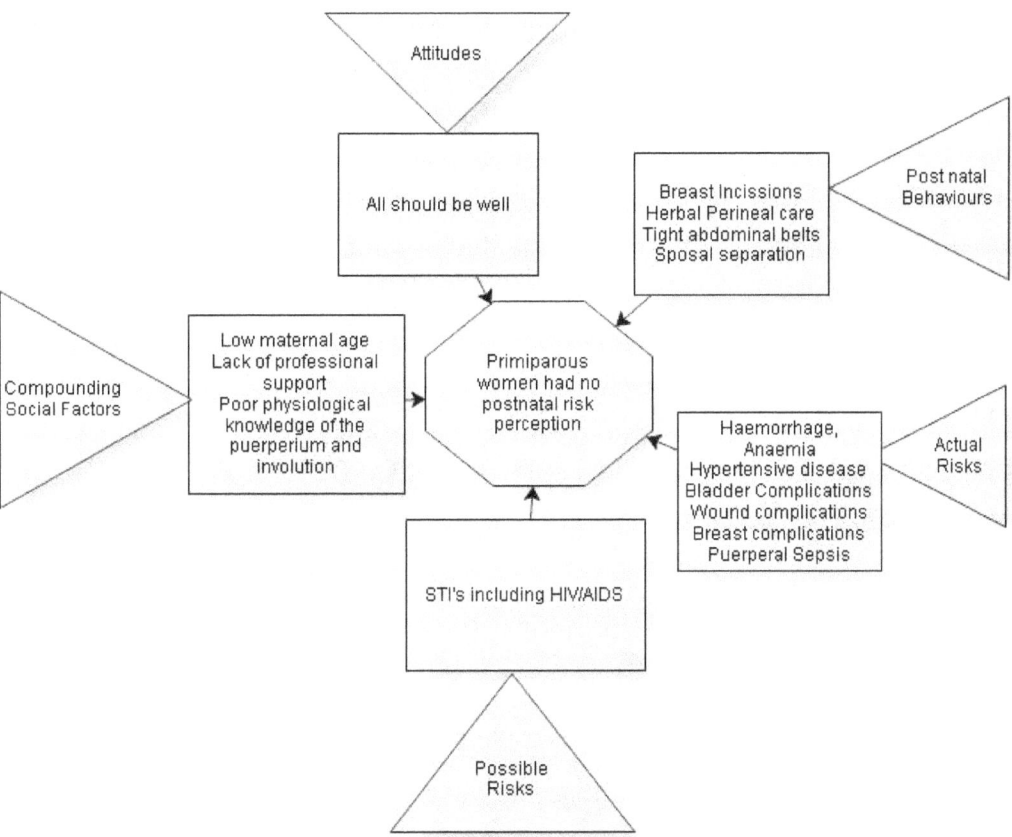

Figure 12.2 Women's Post natal risk perception (Murira,2014).

The concerns and information needs expressed by women in the post natal period, their involvement in and their compliance with some potentially dangerous cultural practices are indications of limited information confirming that primiparous women are likely to have no risk perception at a critical phase in their lives when they have high risk of exposure to morbidity and mortality.

Medical interventions have to be meaningful to health clients in order for them to be accepted and perceived as useful by clients. Interventions can only have meaning to clients if they are fully explained before the event they are intended to prevent, in a language that the clients understand and if these interventions take into consideration what the woman already knows from her culture (Ley, 1988; Leineinger, 2005). Health personnel must have the correct perspective of the women's background, the context and environment in which the cultural practices occur, the women's sources of support, their practices, the aims or goals they intend to achieve through their behaviours, the resources available to the women and the cost of alternatives available to the women to fully understand women's culture.

Unless and until domiciliary post natal visits for women are regarded as an inaugural part of maternal health care and an essential intervention that reduces maternal morbidity and mortality, women will continue to be exposed to perinatal morbidity.

Behavioural Theory

Social cognitive models regard behaviour as emanating from cognitions commonly shared by society (Bandura, 1977, 1986). Social cognition places value and concern of a person on their social world around them. The Theory of Reasoned Action reaffirms that behaviour unfolds within a context influenced by social norms and beliefs(Ajzen & Fishbein,1986). There are several external modifying factors to behaviours in the postnatal period to include socio-cultural factors like what societal or cultural explanation of a problem could be, and if the particular society appreciates one's circumstances and experiences as a problem. The age of an individual is a major behaviour modifier which may affect young inexperienced women's decision- making powers as well as their self-care and baby care skills. First time mothers in many cultures are not regarded as possessing deep understanding and adequate information about life in general let alone reproductive health issues. The elderly family members may see it as their responsibility to control the young women's behaviours from pregnancy until the post natal period. This behaviour is natural and humane and meant to assist the young women to learn gradually through observation but; it is not every mature woman who is well informed with effective health promoting advice and practices. Health personnel should use the postnatal period as a 'teachable period' for women as both community family members and the postnatal mothers are anxious to ensure a speedy recovery of the postnatal mother and are therefore well receptive of health promoting messages during this period(Lawson &Flowke,2008).

The women's culture is carefully planned at each stage of the reproductive phase and follows the Theory of Planned Behaviour (Ajzen, 1980, 1986) at each stage of the woman's reproductive phase from preconception to the post natal period. There are also strong aspects of the Health Belief Model that are highlighted in postnatal behaviours (Rosenstock, 1975; Becker & Maimen, 1980). Elderly women in most societies orchestrate the behaviours of young women with good intentions but the knowledge about each phase of the child bearing process within young women and their mentors and the means that are applied to achieve the intended outcomes may expose some women to risk and morbidity.

Certain social factors such as the level of education, availability of resources, emotion, and perceived symptoms like pain, beliefs of the women and beliefs of the health professionals, have been identified and believed to predict health behaviours (Leventhal et al., 1985). Studies of health behaviours suggest that half of the causes of mortality are due to behaviour and that people's chosen lifestyle and modification of one's health behaviour is the major determinant of one's quality of life. These factors are believed to impact on one's state of health. Awareness of the impact of these factors is believed to delay the onset of ill health (Belloc & Breslow, 1972; Breslow & Enstrom, 1980). This suggests that the health visitor is key to positive community behaviour change through effective health promotion in the families and to individual women and their sources of support.

Research suggests that individuals can make a significant improvement to their lives and enhance their health, increasing longevity through modifying their way of life, by adopting life- enhancing behaviours and avoiding health compromising behaviours. Some of the factors influencing people's health beliefs and behaviour are also social determinants of good health behaviours and these are believed to be good parental models, positive peer influences, positive cultural values, good control of emotional factors, self-esteem and accessibility to health facilities, the impact of social support, area of residence, education and age (Curtis, 2000; Macintyre et al., 2006). Women can be highly influenced and controlled by cultural beliefs and influences to such an extent that all the other determinants of good health can be overruled. In the postnatal period, Murira,(2010) observed that mature women wield a lot of power over a new mother and may ensure that the cultural norms are enforced. This is suggesting and confirming that strong socio-cultural influences and expectations play a major role in women's health behaviour and the state of women's health during the child bearing period. Health personnel cannot hope to influence women's health without addressing women's culture through close monitoring of women post delivery and effective, continuous health promotion efforts.

The impact of fear on women's behaviours

Fear driven by lack of information and belief in reprisals as a result of breach of cultural practices greatly influences women's behaviours. Fear enhances the adoption of cultural practices young women may be instructed to adopt by their mentors. Fear arousing communication is known to influence cognition, attitudes, behavioural intentions and health behaviour (Boer & Seydel, 2003). The Protection motivation theory which extends the Health Belief Model and was developed around the framework of fear arousing communication, explains the impact of fear-laden messages on behaviours (Rogers, 1975; Maddux & Roggers, 1983; Roggers, 1985; Boer & Seydel, 2003). Research suggests that fear arousal does not create consistent behaviour but promotes trial and error behaviour whereas a message with reassuring behavioural advice would reduce threat and fear for one's life. If following advice reduces fear, then the advised behaviour is enhanced, suggesting that health promoting messages can reduce threat of ill health and enable young women to adopt positive health behaviours. The challenge of health personnel is to provide continuous support to women through continuous health messages to women and communities to adopt healthy practices that reduce the temptation to fall back onto ineffective cultural practices.

Adaptive Behaviour

The cognitive reaction of the individual in terms of fear control or danger control is important and essential in adoption of adaptive behaviour (Boer & Seydel, 2003). Enhancing effectiveness of advised behaviour enhances adoption of advised behaviour (Sutton, 1983). Adapting involves assessing the available alternatives to get rid of the threat, an attitude or skill that may be absent in young women.

The adoption of new behaviours and the process of coping with the new behaviour is based on two components; the individual's expectancy that carrying out the action will remove the threat or negative consequences (action-outcome efficacy) and one's capability to put the action into motion (self- efficacy)(Connor & Norman, 2003). Adaptive behaviour seems to occur readily where one perceives the consequences of going against the instructions from a mentor and the fear increases determination to perform the adaptive behaviour. In the presence of health information, a young woman would have an alternative that enables her to make informed choices.

Sources of Information for Adaption

According to the Protection Motivation Theory, there are two sources of information, namely, environmental source that comes in the form of verbal persuasion from significant others; radio, television adverts and observing others perform behaviour. This is called observational learning. The second source of learning is experiential or intra-personal. Young women going through the postnatal period are exposed to both sources of information although the intensity of one source, verbal persuasion from significant others, may dominate the learning process. Where young women receive a lot of information from their cultural mentors and there is no health professional to provide an alternative source of scientific information, young women put the information from their mentors into practice. This is also suggesting that the post natal period is an ideal period for learning for women and health personnel could make a significant impact on women's health by offering information and advice that enhances good health and promotes quick recovery post delivery.

Development of cultural awareness among health personnel enables them to freely interact with women recognizing the women's values and beliefs. Cultural awareness requires that health personnel engage in frequent friendly interaction with women and learn from the women's culture. The elderly women orchestrate the women's behaviours with good intentions but it is the means of achieving the intentions that expose women to the risk of morbidity. It is important that health personnel are at hand in the communities to provide an alternative to cultural teaching and practices.

Individuals can make a significant improvement to their lives and enhance their health, increasing longevity through modifying their way of life, by adopting life- enhancing behaviours and avoiding health compromising behaviours. Parental models, peer influences, cultural values, emotional factors, self-esteem and accessibility to health facilities are some of the social determinants of good health behaviours (Curtis, 2000). The impact of social support, area of residence, education and age are some of the factors influencing people's health beliefs and behaviour (Macintyre et al 2006). Primiparous women can be highly influenced and controlled by culture to such an extent that all the other factors can be overruled. This observation therefore confirms that strong socio-cultural influences and expectations play a major role in women's behaviour during the child bearing process.

Women's Health policy should therefore be led by an objective health needs assessment of women and should address culture as the source of values and cultural health practices (Leineinger, 2005). The focus of health personnel as implementers of policy should be to increase women's opportunities to acquire information, access services of their choice and increase their risk perception. Information should be client centred and phase related to prepare women for subsequent phases along the child bearing process.

It can be concluded that poor quality of communication between health personnel and women may not increase health knowledge in the young primiparous women and may fail to meet the information and self-care needs of the young women. If women fail to access effective information or knowledge throughout the child bearing phases women are likely to display a behaviour that points to lack of knowledge of actual risks they are exposed to and poor understanding of what to expert in each reproductive phase. Women will easily turn to what they know best, what is practised in their communities and will depend heavily on cultural practices within their society some of which may be a source of morbidity.

References

1. Aina,O.I; Adewuyi,A.A; Adesina,Y; Adeyeni,AThe Culture of Male Supremacy and Emergency Obstetric Care: The Nigerian Experience. *The African Anthropologist*, 2002; 136:9(2):157-182

2. Aisien,A.O; Imade,G.E; Sagay,A.S et al., Safety, Efficacy and Acceptability of Norplant Implants in Jos, Northern Nigeria. *Tropical Journal of Obstetrics and Gynaecology*, 2004;21 (2): 42-49

3. Ajzen,I; Fishbein,M)*Understanding attitudes and predicting social behaviour*. Englewood Cliffs,1980. NJ: Prentice Hall

4. Balaskas, J.. *Active Birth. Unwin Paperbacks*, 1989. London.

5. *Bandura, A.* Social Learning Theory. *Englewood Cliffs. Prentice Hall, 1977. N.J.*

6. *Bandura, A.* Social Foundations of Thought and Action. *Eaglewood- Cliffs, 1986. N.J.*

7. Barnett,B;Konate,M;Mhloyi,M et al.,The impact of family Planning on Women's lives: Findings from the Women's Studies Project in Mali and Zimbabwe. *African Journal of Reproductive Health*, 1999; 49:3 (1): 75-81

8. Becker,M.H. The Health Belief Model and personal health behaviour. *Health Education Monograms*, 1975; 2 (4):115-7

9. Becker, M.H; Maiman, L.A. *Models of health-related behaviour*. In D. Mechanic (ed). Handbook of Health, Health Care and the Health Professions. Free Press, 1983. New York.

10. Belloc, N. B; Breslow, L. Relationship of physical health status and health practices, *Preventive Medicine*,1972;9: 409-421

11. Boer, H; Seydel,E.R. *Protection Motivation Theory*. In Conner, M. and Norman, P. Predicting Health Behaviour. Open University Press, 2005. Bucking.

12. Breslow, L; Enstrom, J.E. Persistence of health habits and their relationship to mortality. *Preventive Medicine*,1980; 9: 469-83

13. Bryar, R.M. *Theory for Midwifery Practice*. Macmillan Publishing,1995. London

14. Brookfield,S.D. Undesternding and Facilitating Adult Learning. Open Univesity Press. 1986. Milton Keynes

15. Conner, M; Norman, P. *Protection Motivation Theory*. In Predicting Health Behaviour. Open University Press, 2005. Bucking

16. Conner, M; Norman, P. *Predicting Health Behaviour*. Open University Press, 2005. Bucking.

17. Curtis, A.J. *Health Psychology*. Routledge, 2000. London.

18. Dow, T.E. Jr and Werner, L.H. (1981). Family size and Family Planning in Kenya: Continuity and change in metropolitan and rural attitudes. *Studies in Family Planning*. 12(6-7), pp. 272-277.

19. Ekabua,J; Agan,T.U; Etuk,S.J et al., The profile of Norplant Acceptors in Calabar. *Mary Slessor Journal of Medicine*, 2004; 4 (1):75-79

20. Ellis, C. (1995). Doctor-Patient Relationship. *S.A. Family Practice*. 3, pp. 187-191.

21. Epstein, R.M. Making communication research matter: What do patients notice, what do patients want, and what do patients need? *Patient Education and Counselling*, 2006; 60: 272-278

22. Ewles,L; Simnett,I. *Promoting health: a practice guide*. 4th ed. Bailliere Tindall, 1999. Edinburgh

23. Glaister K; Michael M. Patient Health Education Literature. International *Journal of Health Promotion and Education,* 2006; 44(2):83-88

24. Graham, A., Moore, L., Sharp, D. and Diamond, I. (2004). Improving teenagers' knowledge of emergency contraception. Cluster randomized trial of teacher led intervention. *BMJ*. 324, pp. 1179.

25. Helman, C.G.. *Culture, Health and Illness* 4th Ed. Arnold-Hodder, 2001. London

26. Hunter, L. (2008). Teenagers' experiences of postnatal care and breastfeeding. *British Journal of Midwifery*. 16(12), pp. 785-790.

27. Jewell, S.E. Patient Participation: What does it mean to nurses? *Journal of Advanced Nursing,*1994; 19: 433-438

28. Kabir,M; Iliyasu,Z; Abubakar,I. et al., The role of men in contraceptive decision-making in Fanshekara Village, Northern Nigeria. *Tropical Journal of Obstertrics and Gynaecology,* 2003; 20 (1): 23-29

29. Katz, V.L. Maternal Mortality. The correct Assessment Is Everything. *Obstetrics and Gynaecology,* 2005; 106 (4)Editorial

30. Kavanagh,K.H; Kennedy,P.H. Promoting Cultural Diversity. *Sage Publications,* 1992. CA.

31. Lee C. *Women's Health: Psychological and Social Perspectives*. Sage Publications, 1998. California.

32. Leininger,M.M; McFarland,M.R. *Culture Care Diversity and Universality. A Worldwide Nursing Theory*. 2nd. Ed. Jones & Bartlett Publishers, 2006. London

33. Leininger, M.M. Theoretical Questions and Concerns: Response from the Theory of Culture Care Diversity and Universality Perspective. *Nursing Science Quarterly,* 2007;20(9): 9-13

34. Leventhal, H; Nerez,D.R; Steel, D.F. *Illness representations and coping with health threats*. In Baum, A; Singer, A. Handbook of Psychology and Health,1984. Hillsdale, NJ

35. Ley, P. *Communicating with Patients: Improving Communication, Satisfaction, and Compliance*. Croom Helm, 1988. London.

36. Lupton, D. *RISK*. Routledge,1999. London and New York

37. Macintyre,S; McKay,L; Ellaway,A. Lay concepts of the relative importance of different influences on health; are there major socio-demographic variations? *Health Education Research Theory and Practice*, 2006; 21 (5):731-736

38. Maddux, J.E; Rogers,R.W. Protection Motivation and self-efficacy: a revised theory of fear appeals and attitude change. *Journal of Experimental Social Psychology,* 1983; 19: 469-79

39. Madebwe, C. and Madebwe, V. (2006). Post marital return to natal home to have the first birth: does this socio-cultural tradition disempower women? Evidence from Gweru, Zimbabwe. *East African Social Science Research Review*. 22(2), pp. 51-64.Mesfin,GThe role of men in fertility and family planning program in Tigray Region. *Ethiopian Journal of Health Development,* 2002;16(3) : 247-255

40. Murira,N. Communicating Sexual and Reproductive Health messages. PhD Thesis. Birmingham City University, (2010).Centre for Health and Social Care Research

41. Naidoo, J; Wills, J. *Health Promotion*. Foundations for Practice.2nd Ed.Bailliere Tindall, 2004. Edinburgh

42. Rosenstock, I.R. *The Health Belief Model: Explaining Health Behaviour through expectancies*. In K. Glantnz (Ed) Health behaviour and health education: theory, research, and practice, Jossey-Bass, San Francisco, 1990: 39-62

43. Sanogo,D; RamaRao, S; Jones,H et al., Improving Quality of Care and Use of Contraceptives in Senegal. *African Journal of Reproductive Health,* 2003; 7 (2) 57-73

44. Sutton, S.R. *Fear Arousing Communications: a critical examination of theory and research.* In J.R. Eiser (ed). Social Psychology and Behavioural Medicine. London: Wiley, 1982: 307-37.

45. Tanvatanakul, V; Amado, J; Saowakontha, S. Management of communication channels for health information in the community. *Health Education Journal,* 2007; 66(2):173-178

Index